Dax's Case

Dax's Case

Essays in Medical Ethics and Human Meaning

EDITED BY LONNIE D. KLIEVER

Southern Methodist University Press

First Edition, 1989
Requests for permission to reproduce material from this work
should be sent to:

Rights and Permissions
Southern Methodist University Press
Box 415
Dallas, Texas 75275

Library of Congress Cataloging-in-Publication Data
Dax's case.
Includes index.
1. Cowart, Donald—Health.   2. Burns and scalds—
Patients—United States—Biography.   3. Burns and
scalds—Treatment—Moral and ethical aspects.   4. Medical care—Moral
and ethical aspects.   I. Kliever, Lonnie D.
RD96.4.C69D38   1988   362.1'97'110924   [B] 88-42636
ISBN 0-87074-277-9
ISBN 0-87074-278-7 (pbk.)

Grateful acknowledgment is made for permission to reprint the following:

Excerpt from *J. B.: A Play in Verse* by Archibald MacLeish.
Copyright © 1956, 1957, 1958 by Archibald MacLeish.
Copyright © 1986 by William H. MacLeish and Mary Grimm.
Reprinted by permission of Houghton Mifflin Company.

Excerpt from Gilgamesh Epic, cited in *Ancient Myth and Modern Life*
by Gerald A. Larue, published by Center Line Press.
Translation used by permission of Gerald A. Larue.

Excerpt from *A Masque of Reason* by Robert Frost.
Copyright © 1945 by Robert Frost.
Reprinted by permission of Henry Holt and Company.

FOR DAX COWART

Contents

CONTENTS

Preface

DONALD "DAX" COWART IS A SURVIVOR OF A PRO-
pane gas explosion in the summer of 1973 that left him totally
blind, permanently disfigured, and severely maimed. Despite his
massive handicaps, he now lives a reasonably comfortable and productive life. He is financially secure by virtue of an out-of-court
settlement with the energy company whose leaking pipeline caused
the accident. He recently graduated from law school and has set up
a small legal practice in his hometown of Henderson, Texas. But,
had Dax Cowart been given his way, he would have never survived
his horrifying ordeal. Through fourteen long months of painful
treatment in three different hospitals, he repeatedly demanded that
he be allowed to die. He pled with his mother and lawyer to be
discharged from the hospital. He raged against the treatment his
doctors and therapists provided. But neither his family nor his physicians would consent to his demands. He remained in the hospital
and received treatment until he was well enough to be released to his
mother's care. Thereafter, he languished through years of virtual
helplessness until he finally began to build a new personal identity
and public life for himself. Though his efforts have been successful
beyond anyone's expectations, he remains convinced to this day that
he should have been allowed to die.

As such, Cowart's story presents a remarkable "case study" of a whole range of life-or-death issues that challenge professionals in a number of fields and confront individuals in every walk of life. Care for the hopelessly ill and the severely handicapped raises medical, legal, and moral problems of the greatest complexity for practitioners in medicine, law, and the ministry. What are the dividing lines between life and death? Where are the limits on life-supporting and death-postponing medical treatment? Who are the parties responsible for making treatment decisions for the suffering and the dying? The Cowart case raises these questions in bold relief precisely because he was fully capable of making an informed and reflective decision about continuing or discontinuing his treatment. But his repeated demands to die were dismissed by family and physicians alike as little more than dramatic protests against his painful treatment, helpless condition, and foreboding future. Those naked conflicts between patient, family, and physician reveal more clearly than most life-or-death treatment situations that competing values, conflicting interests, and clashing powers are at the heart of all such circumstances.

For similar reasons, the Cowart story confronts ordinary individuals with the deepest questions concerning life's meaning and purpose. Experiences of great confusion, suffering, or tragedy are always a threat to feelings of personal security and well-being. Individuals or groups overtaken by such experiences typically look to the consolations of philosophy or the reassurances of religion to restore some sense of the world's dependable regularity, moral coherence, and transcendent purpose. But the Cowart case takes us to the very limits of human understanding, endurance, and purpose. Shallow philosophies and superficial religions are strained to the breaking point by the questions that Cowart's ordeal forces on us. Where are the final boundaries of individual freedom and social responsibility? What are the ultimate sources of human comfort and consolation? How can life finally go on in the face of overwhelming handicaps and unrelenting misery? Moreover, Cowart's experience reminds us of the precariousness of our everyday routines, ordinary capabilities, and cherished expectations. These foundations of life can be taken away in a moment of catastrophic accident or gradually wasted away through the ravages of a lingering illness. Whatever the circumstance, human life is always a triumph over the threatened loss of the very things that give meaning and purpose to life.

The essays in this volume explore this entire range of issues. Coming from a variety of disciplines and professions, the authors approach Dax's "case" with very different questions from very different perspectives. For some, the Cowart story is a definitive example of the unresolved conflicts between patient rights and professional duties that surround the entire health care system. Cowart's ordeal illuminates the profound dilemmas that arise when a patient, family, and health care staff disagree on treatment decisions and moral issues. For others, the Cowart story is a vivid documentation of the inherent tensions between social institutions and personal values. Cowart's experience reveals the ways in which institutions designed to maximize human safety and security, health and happiness may run counter to the express convictions and desires of certain individuals served by those institutions. Still for others, the Cowart story is a powerful metaphor for rethinking the myths and rituals by which societies and individuals deal with life's absurdities. Cowart's struggle with life and death exposes the fragile boundaries and the stubborn alliances between danger and creativity, between suffering and beatitude. By thus reviewing Dax's case, these varied essays bring into clearer view the narrowest problems in medical ethics and the broadest questions of human meaning.

Cowart's ordeal would have never become a celebrated "case study" in medical ethics and human meaning had his story not been told in two remarkable films. The first film is a thirty-minute videotape, entitled *Please Let Me Die*, which was produced in the late spring of 1974 as an in-house teaching instrument for the medical faculty at the University of Texas Medical Branch in Galveston. The videotape features an interview of Cowart by Dr. Robert B. White, professor of psychiatry, concerning his wish to die. Cowart had been transferred to the Galveston hospital's critical care burn unit from the Texas Institute for Research and Rehabilitation in Houston, where he had recently begun a rehabilitative care program following eight months of treatment at Parkland Hospital in Dallas. While in Houston, Cowart's burn wounds had become seriously reinfected as a result of his refusing treatment and demanding discharge from that hospital. Upon his arrival in Galveston, Cowart's primary care physician requested a psychiatric evaluation by Dr. White to see if his wish to die was the result of some emotional illness or mental aberration. White found that Cowart was fully able to make a rational and informed decision about accepting or refusing treatment. In fact, he was so impressed with the clarity and forcefulness of Cowart's demands to die that he arranged for a videotape of this unique clash between patient's rights and physician's duties.

Viewing *Please Let Me Die* is a memorable though unsettling experience, even for the medical professionals for whom it was originally made. The videotape vividly depicts the debridement process, an extremely painful procedure wherein burn victims have dead tissue and dressing remnants scraped off their wounds daily. Cowart is shown being bathed in a large whirlpool filled with a warm water and chlorox solution. Following the "tanking," masked attendants gently apply medicated gauzes to Cowart's burn wounds amid intermittent screams of pain and protest. The camera pans from his emaciated body to close-up shots of his raw wounds, his maimed hands, his scarred face, his graft-covered eye socket. In sharp contrast to these horrific treatment scenes, Cowart later lies quietly in his bed and responds in measured voice to White's gentle questioning about his reasons for wanting to die. He explains at some length why he does not want to go on living as a blind and crippled person. He had led a full and active life as a high school athlete and air force jet pilot. He had loved the outdoors and enjoyed the party scene. The pain of his treatment was so great and the prospects of his rehabilitation were so small that death seemed the only sensible and decent option open to him. And yet that option was being denied him by his family and physicians. *Please Let*

Me Die closes with Cowart's survival and recovery very much in question.

Although not intended for general distribution, *Please Let Me Die* became a "classic" among professionals concerned with the treatment and care of the hopelessly ill and the helplessly deformed. It was periodically shown at professional society meetings around the world and regularly used for classroom instruction at medical, law, and divinity schools. But, for all of its powerful imagery and eloquent argument, the videotape is limited in two significant ways. *Please Let Me Die* presents only one side of the issues raised by this remarkable case. Cowart's account of his uncaring treatment by others and his unwavering demands to die are neither challenged nor confirmed by others who were involved in his care. His mother and lawyer, his doctors and nurses are not given an opportunity to explain their interpretation of Cowart's behavior and their unwillingness to let him die. Moreover, *Please Let Me Die* ends with many of the questions that it raises left unanswered. What happened to Cowart after his filmed interview with White? Did he persist in his efforts to gain his release from the hospital? Did he survive his harrowing ordeal despite his desire to die? Has he made a successful adjustment to his massive handicaps? Has he found reason to be glad that he survived? Viewers of the videotape are left wondering whether Cowart was successful in his efforts to refuse treatment or whether Cowart eventually changed his mind about wanting to die.

The second film, entitled *Dax's Case,* was expressly produced to reach a wider audience with a fuller telling of the Cowart story. In the fall of 1979, a free-lance journalist named Keith Burton had seen *Please Let Me Die* in a bioethics seminar at Southern Methodist University. He was intrigued by the untold story and the unanswered questions in the videotape and decided to learn more about this remarkable man. He managed to contact Cowart and his mother in the spring of 1980 and won their interest in the possibility of a film updating the videotape. Burton enlisted the help of Don Pasquella, an SMU professor of cinematography, and the two of them spent a year seeking financial support from public and private foundations. The Texas Committee for the Humanities expressed strong interest in the project, but their promised grant was far short of the money needed. Eventually Concern for Dying, a highly respected New York educational council in the field of death and dying, agreed to develop and produce the film with Burton and Pasquella's assistance. Concern for Dying spent another two years in fundraising and background research for the film while the film's actual production took an additional year and a half. *Dax's Case* was finally released in 1985 and won that year's Runner-Up Award in the feature-length "Social Issues" category of the American Film Festival.

Dax's Case tracks the Cowart story from the summer of 1973 to the fall of 1984. Opening shots place a rustically dressed Cowart at the scene of the accident, explaining the explosion and its aftermath. His scarred flesh and maimed body are eloquent testimony to the horrors that he has endured. Viewers of the film instinctively understand why Cowart was so eager to die. His survival was achieved at a cost of personal pain and loss almost beyond imagination. Cowart later appears on camera, impeccably dressed and sitting in his own plush office, where he thoughtfully muses about patient rights and free choice. Just as quickly, viewers of the film understand why his family and physicians would not let him die. Cowart obviously has the personal abilities and the financial resources to make something of his life despite his physical limitations. The remainder of the film explores this clash of perspectives and sentiments through vivid scenes and conflicting interpretations of Cowart's accident, treatment, and rehabilitation. All the principal figures in this remarkable life-and-death drama are given the chance to speak their minds. Cowart makes his case for wanting to die while his loved ones and caretakers explain why they were unwilling to grant his desires. The film ends without final resolution—Cowart insisting that he should have been allowed to die even though his life now is not without rewards, Cowart's mother, lawyer, and physicians acknowledging his profound suffering but deeply gratified that he was not allowed to die.

Obviously, *Dax's Case* was designed primarily for classroom use. The film, which is available for rental or purchase from Concern for Dying, is widely used in training medical, legal, and ministerial professionals and in teaching undergraduates in the humanities and social sciences. Its narrative form enables viewers to relive the complexities of such medical and legal decisions, the divergences of such moral and religious commitments for themselves. Its interrogative tone compels viewers to ponder the limits of freedom and responsibility, the meaning of life and death. In keeping with these pedagogical purposes, the Texas Committee for the Humanities and Concern for Dying provided matching supplemental grants for the preparation of this volume for use in conjunction with the film. But, though written expressly as responses to *Dax's Case*, these essays transcend the film in two important ways. Understanding the essays does not totally depend upon having seen the film. An introductory "Chronicle" by Keith Burton and "Memoir" by Robert B. White clearly establish the historical and medical context of Cowart's accident, treatment, and rehabilitation. Nor are the essays limited to a discussion of the Cowart story per se. Each author seeks out the wider issues and develops the fuller implications of the Cowart story from their own particular disciplinary points of view. For these reasons, this volume should prove valuable not only as extended commentaries on the film *Dax's Case* but also as provocative meditations on human life at the edges of endurance and the limits of hope.

Lonnie D. Kliever
Dallas, 1988

Dax's Case

A Chronicle: Dax's Case As It Happened 🔯 *Keith Burton*

WHEN I WAS A BOY, DEATH WAS NOT AN ENEMY. ITS presence brought peace and new beginnings—feelings I still connect with when remembering my grandfather's death twenty-five years ago: He was buried on a cold November day. A bitter wind forced us to huddle closely together near the casket. The preacher comforted us with final remarks at the open grave. In the winter sky, the setting sun bathed wispy clouds in crimson red. Grief gave way to a peaceful release. These are the images remembered.

My own feelings about death occupied me as I drove on toward the causeway bridge linking Galveston Island to Texas. The date was April 19, 1980. Five months earlier, in a bioethics course at Southern Methodist University, I had viewed a videotape about a man named Donald Cowart who had been severely burned in a 1973 propane gas explosion in East Texas. Cowart had sought to refuse the medical treatment that saved his life. The videotape, *Please Let Me Die*, had become a living record of this man's struggle for release from pain and despair. But the videotape left me wondering whatever happened to that man. My journey in search of Cowart had taken me to Galveston, where I would meet him for the first time.

The story of Don Cowart is remarkable in some ways but

commonplace in others. A man's wish to die is rather extraordinary in and of itself; but the pattern of events that shape such a wish often is woven of the fabric of life's everyday occurrences. Such is the case with Cowart.

Ray and Ada Cowart moved their family from the Rio Grande Valley to the small East Texas town of Henderson in the sixties. Ray prospered over the years as a rancher and real estate agent. Ada became a teacher in the Henderson school district. Their three children—Don, Jim, and Beth—were no different from other kids reared in a close-knit community. In fact, they were ordinary people living ordinary lives.

"Donny Boy," as he came to be called by his father, was popular in school and excelled in athletics. He was captain of his high school football team and performed in rodeos. He liked to take risks, a trait that often dismayed his mother. It was risk taking that would later lure him to skydiving, surfing, and other sports of chance.

Don Cowart left Henderson in 1966 to attend the University of Texas at Austin. He had planned to return home at his graduation three years later to join his father in business; however, when notified of his military draft selection, Cowart instead elected to join the U.S. Air Force. He became a pilot and served in Vietnam. He married a high school sweetheart in 1972, but they divorced eight months later. In May 1973 he was discharged from active duty and returned to Henderson, where he began working with his father in real estate.

Life back in East Texas brought Cowart warmth and new independence in the summer of 1973. It was a quiet summer. Now twenty-five years old, he had returned home to decide the future course of his career. He had several options—to become a commercial airline pilot, to join his father as a real estate broker, or to attend law school. And he was dating again after having endured the breakup of his first marriage. The new relationship seemed promising.

July 23, 1973, seemed no different to Cowart from any other

Wednesday. It was hot and sultry as the afternoon sun slipped low along the pine trees in the countryside near Henderson. Ray and Don had driven out to a ranch to look over some property being offered for sale by the owner. They parked their car on a bridge over a dry creek and took off by foot. They talked and laughed together as they surveyed points of interest on the land. Their business completed, the Cowarts then returned to their car to go home for dinner.

Ada Cowart didn't think it odd that her husband and son were late arriving home. Sometimes Ray's business dealings delayed him in the evenings. She went about preparing the meal and sat down with her daughter to eat. They turned on the radio to catch the news. Ada remembers hearing a report of an explosion and fire in the oil fields which had injured two men outside Henderson. The names of the injured had not been given. All that was known was one man was critically injured, the other seriously injured.

Wednesday was church night for the Cowarts. Though Ray and Don still hadn't arrived home, Ada went on to services without them. She was in class studying a Bible lesson when the police chief and Ray Cowart's secretary arrived at the door asking for her. There had been an explosion, Ada was told, and Ray and Don were badly hurt. The extent of their injuries remained unknown. It was then that the earlier radio report flashed back into her mind in horrifying fashion.

The accident happened with no warning. The Cowart men had returned to their car but had not been able to start the engine. Ray had lifted the hood and removed the air cleaner from the engine. He primed the carburetor by hand and instructed Don to try the ignition. Several tries failed. It seemed to Don that the battery was near exhaustion. A final attempt proved fateful, however, as a blue flame shot from the carburetor and ignited a terrible explosion and fire.

Ray Cowart was hurled into heavy underbrush by the force of the explosion. The blast rocked the car and showered window glass over Don's body. Around them, the fireball spread quickly, consuming pine trees and the scrub vegetation in the area. Don reacted quickly. He climbed from the burning car and began running toward the woods. But he was forced to stop by a fear that he would become entangled in the underbrush and slowly burn to death.

Don wheeled about and decided to chance the dirt road on which they had driven in. He ran through three walls of fire, emerged into a clearing, then fell to the ground and rolled his body to extinguish the flames. He got back to his feet and resumed running in search of help for his father.

It all seemed dreamlike. Don noticed his vision was blurred as though swimming under water. His eyes had been badly burned. Now the pain was coming in waves, and he knew it was real. He kept running.

Loud voices filtered through the woods. Don collapsed at the roadside as help arrived. He heard the footsteps of a man and then the exclamation, "Oh, my God!" when a farmer found him. Don sent the man after his father and lay wondering how badly he was burned. When the man returned, Don asked him to bring a gun— a gun he would use to kill himself. The farmer refused.

In shock, Don assumed he and his father had caused the explosion by igniting gasoline from the car's engine. Later he would learn that the explosion actually had been caused by a leaking propane gas transmission line in the area where they had parked. It was a freak event. A pocket of propane gas had formed in the dry creekbed. When the carburetor flamed up, it had ignited the gas.

Rescuers took the Cowart men to a hospital in nearby Kilgore. There, a decision was made to transport them by ambulance to a special burn unit at Dallas's Parkland Hospital. Ray Cowart died en route to Dallas. Don Cowart remembers incredible pain, his begging for pain medication, and the paramedic's refusal to administer drugs prior to their arrival in Dallas. By this time, Ada Cowart, too, was on her way to Dallas. She had returned home first to pack several changes of clothes. The radio had said the men were badly hurt. She didn't expect to return to Henderson any time soon.

Even as the ambulance sped the 140 miles from Kilgore to

Dallas, Don Cowart's treatment regimen had begun. By telephone, Dr. Charles Baxter, head of Parkland's burn unit, had directed fluid therapies to help in preventing shock to vital organs. On examination in Dallas, Baxter found Cowart had severe burns over 65 percent of his body. His face suffered third-degree burns and both eyes were severely damaged. His ears and hands were also deeply burned. Fluid therapies continued and were aided by several other measures: the insertion of an intertracheal tube to control the airway, catheters placed in every body opening, treatment with antibiotics, cleansing the wounds with antibacterial drugs, and tetanus prophylaxis. Heavy doses of narcotics were given for the pain.

In the early days of Don's 232-day hospitalization at Parkland, doctors could not predict whether he would survive. It was touch and go for many weeks. Ada Cowart felt helpless; she could do little more than sit in the waiting area outside the intensive care unit with relatives of other burn victims, where she prayed and hoped for the best. Doctors permitted only short visits with her son. Don had given his mother power of attorney in the Parkland emergency room, and she in turn deferred to the medical professionals on treatment decisions.

For Cowart, there were countless whirlpool tankings in solutions to cleanse his wounds; procedures to remove dead tissue, grafts to protect living tissue, the amputation of badly charred fingers from both hands and the removal of his right eye. The damaged left eye was sewn shut. And there was terrible pain.

Through it all, Don had remained constant in his view that he did not want to live. His demands to die had started with the farmer at the accident site. They had continued at the Kilgore hospital, in the ambulance, and now at Parkland. He didn't want treatment that would extend his misery and he made this known to his mother and family, Dr. Charles Baxter, a nurse named Leslie Kerr, longtime friend Art Rousseau, attorney Rex Houston, and many others.

Baxter remained undaunted by Don's pleas to stop treatment, dismissing them at first as the typical response of burn victims to the pain of their wounds and treatment. In time, however, he openly discussed Cowart's wish to die with Don, his mother, and lawyer, considering all the medical and legal ramifications. Failing to get Ada Cowart's and Rex Houston's consent to the withdrawal of treatment, Baxter continued to deliver it.

For her part, Ada Cowart understood her son's pain and anguish. She was haunted, nonetheless, by these thoughts: What if treatment were ceased and Don changed his mind in a near-death state? Would it be too late? Furthermore, her religious beliefs simply made mercy killing or suicide deplorable options. These religious constraints were reinforced by her fear that her son had not yet made his "peace with God."

Rex Houston also had mixed feelings about Don's wishes. On the one hand, he sympathized with Cowart's condition—being unable to so much as take medication to end his life without the assistance of others. On the other hand, it was Houston's duty to reach a favorable resolution of a lawsuit filed against the pipeline owners for Ray Cowart's death and for Don Cowart's disability. With regard to the latter, he needed a living plaintiff to achieve the best damage award for the Cowart family. Moreover, Houston believed that such an award would provide the financial means necessary for Don Cowart's ultimate rehabilitation. He therefore encouraged Cowart to see the legal proceedings through.

In February 1974, the lawsuit was settled out of court—one day prior to trial. Almost immediately, Don's demands to die quickened. There had been talk before with Art Rousseau of getting a gun. Don had asked Leslie Kerr if she would help him by injecting an overdose of medication. Now Cowart even talked with Houston about helping him get to a window of his sixth-floor hospital room, where presumably he would leap to his death. All listened but none agreed to help.

On March 12, 1974, Don was discharged from Parkland. He, his family, and doctors agreed that his condition had improved sufficiently to warrant his transfer to the Texas Institute for Research and Rehabilitation in Houston. Nine months removed from his medical residency, Dr. Robert Meier of TIRR found Cowart to be a passive recipient of medical care, although the philosophy of treatment in this rehabilitation center encouraged patient involvement in treatment decisions. Previously Don had no say in his care; now he would be offered choices in his own treatment.

All seemed to go well during the first three weeks of his stay, until Cowart realized the pain he had endured might continue indefinitely, thanks to a careless comment by a resident plastic surgeon that his treatment would be years in completion. Faced with that prospect, Cowart refused treatment for his open burn areas and stopped taking food and water. In a matter of days, Cowart's medical condition deteriorated rapidly. Finding his patient in serious condition, Dr. Meier was deeply perplexed about what do do next. He believed it his duty to help Cowart achieve the highest measure of rehabilitation, but he was not inclined to force upon the patient care he did not wish to receive. Faced with this dilemma, he called for a meeting with Ada Cowart and Rex Houston to discuss with Don the future course of his treatment.

Ada Cowart was outraged by Don's condition. She had been discouraged from staying with her son at TIRR, and in her absence his burns had worsened. He was again near death, due to his refusal of whirlpool tankings and dressing changes. It was agreed in the meeting that Cowart would be transferred to the burn unit of John Sealy Hospital of the University of Texas Medical Branch in Galveston, where his injuries could again be treated by burn specialists.

On April 15, 1974, Don was admitted to the Galveston hospital, in chronic distress from infected wounds, poor nutrition, and severe depression. His right elbow and right wrist were locked tight. The stubs of his fingers on both hands were encased in grotesque skin "mittens." There was practically no skin on his legs. His right eye socket and closed left eye oozed infection. And excruciating pain remained his constant nemesis.

Active wound care was initiated immediately and further skin grafts were advised by Dr. Duane Larson to heal the open wounds on Cowart's chest, legs, and arms. But Cowart bitterly protested the daily tankings and refused to consent to surgery. One night he even crawled out of bed, hoping to throw himself through the window to his death, but he was discovered on the floor and returned to bed.

Frustrated by Cowart's behavior, Dr. Larson consulted Dr. Robert White of psychiatric services for an evaluation of Don's mental competency. White remembers being puzzled by Cowart: Was he a man who tolerated discomfort poorly or perhaps was profoundly depressed? Or was this an extraordinary man who had undergone such an incredible ordeal that he was frustrated beyond normal limits? White concluded, and a colleague confirmed, that Cowart was certainly not mentally incompetent. In fact, he was so impressed with the clarity of Cowart's expressed wish to die that he asked permission to do a videotape interview for classroom use in presenting the medical, ethical, and legal problems surrounding such cases. That filmed interview, which White entitled *Please Let Me Die*, eventually became a classic on patient rights in the field of medical ethics.

Having been declared mentally competent, Cowart still found it difficult to gain control over his treatment. He and his mother argued constantly over treatment procedures. Rex Houston helped get changes in his wound care but turned a deaf ear to Cowart's plea to go home to die from his wounds or to take his own life. In desperation, Cowart turned to other family members for assistance in securing legal representation, but without success. Finally, with White's help, Cowart reached an attorney who had represented Jehovah's Witnesses in their efforts to refuse medical treatment, but he was not optimistic that a lawsuit would free him from the hospital.

Rebuffed on every hand, Cowart reluctantly became more cooperative. White secured changes in Don's pain medication before and after the daily tankings, making treatments more bearable. Psychotherapy and medication helped improve his overall outlook by relieving his depression and improving his sleep. Encouraged that he might still regain sight in his left eye, Don more or less accepted his daily wound care and even agreed to surgical skin grafts early in June 1974. By July 15, his physical condition had improved

enough to allow him to transfer out of the burn unit of the John
Sealy Hospital to the psychiatric unit of the Jennie Sealy Hospital in
the University of Texas Medical Branch under White's direct care
while his wounds continued to heal.

Amid these changes there were still periodic conflicts between
Cowart and those around him over his confinement in the hospital.
There were reiterated demands to die and protests against treatment.
A particularly explosive encounter between Cowart and Larson occurred on the day preceding his second and last major surgical procedure in the Galveston hospital. Cowart had agreed to undergo
surgery to free up his hands, but the night before he changed his
mind. The next morning, Larson angrily confronted Cowart with
the challenge that, if he really wanted to die, he would agree to
the surgery that would enable him to leave the hospital and go
home where he could take his own life if he wished. Anxious to do
exactly that, Cowart consented to the surgery which was performed
on July 31.

Don Cowart's stormy stay at Galveston finally ended on September 19, 1974. He had been hospitalized for a total of fourteen
months, but at last he was going home. His prognosis upon dis-
missal was listed simply as "guarded."

Cowart was glad to be back in Henderson. The little things
counted the most—sleeping in his own bed, listening to music, vis-
iting with friends. But it was different for him than before the accident. He was totally blind, his left eye having failed to recover. His
hands and arms remained useless. He was badly scarred. A dropped
foot now required that someone assist him in walking. Some of his
burn sites still were not healed.

Everything he did required the help of others. Someone had
to feed him, bathe him, and help with personal functions. The days
seemed endless. He tried to find peace in sleep, but even this dark release was impossible without drugs. While he couldn't see himself,
Don knew his appearance drew whispers and stares in restaurants.

He had his tapes, talking books, television, and CB radio. He
could use his sense of hearing, though not as well as before due to

the explosion and burns. And he could think. For a while, he could see in his mind's eye the memories of earlier times. Then the memories started to fade.

Ada Cowart had lost much, but she never lost her religious faith. There had been times when even she had admitted that maybe it would have been best if Don had died with her husband. She reconciled her doubt with the thought that no mother can give up the life of a son. Ada never gave up hope that Don could find new faith in God.

Homecoming brought peace for a time. As Don's early excitement for returning home gave way to deep depression and despair, however, conflict returned to their lives. They argued about how he could occupy himself, how he dressed, his personal habits, and his future. Frustration led to a veiled suicide attempt, Don stealing away from the house during the night to try throwing himself in the path of trucks hauling clay to a brick plant. The police found him and brought him home quietly.

For the next five years, Cowart lived in a shadow world of painful rehabilitation, chronic boredom, and failed relationships. His difficulties were not for want of trying. With Rex Houston's encouragement and assistance he tried pursuing a law degree. Fortunately, his legal settlement with the pipeline company provided the financial means for the nursing care and tutorial assistance which would be required because of his massive handicaps.

Cowart tested out his abilities as a blind student in two undergraduate courses at the University of Texas in Austin during the fall of 1975. He spent the spring at home in Henderson preparing for the tests that were required for admission to law school. In the summer of 1976, he enrolled for a part-time course load in Baylor University's School of Law.

Don handled his studies at Baylor in fine fashion despite his handicaps, but the strain was tremendous. He was forced to live with other people, his independence was limited, and his sleep problems persisted. When a special relationship with a woman ended abruptly in the spring of 1977, his life caved in. He tried to commit suicide by taking an overdose of pain and sleep medications, but he was discovered in time to have his stomach pumped at the hospital emergency room. He had trouble picking up his studies again, so he dropped out before the spring quarter was completed.

Cowart returned home defeated and discouraged, living with his mother for the next half year. He resumed his studies at Baylor in the spring of 1978, only to drop out again before he had completed the third quarter in the fall of 1979. He again retreated to his mother's home, filled with doubts that he would ever be able to pass the bar. By the spring of 1980, he was ready for another try at schooling, this time in a graduate program in building construction at Texas A&M University. Once again, the old patterns of sleepless nights and boring days got the best of him and he made a half-hearted effort at slashing his wrists with a razor blade.

Looking back, Cowart saw his futile efforts to take his own life as a bitter human comedy. The doctors in Galveston had encouraged him to accept treatment that would free him of hospitalization and permit him to end his life, if that was his wish. But he found it difficult to find a way of killing himself without bringing further misery on himself—brain damage or further hospitalization. Ironically, he realized that he was no more successful in ending his life than in making his life work.

As a last resort, Cowart contacted White for help and was voluntarily readmitted under White's care to the Jennie Sealy Hospital on April 12, 1980. During his month-long stay, he met with White for psychotherapy treatments daily. Even more important, his sleep problems were finally resolved by weaning him away from the heavy sleep medications that he had taken for years. Cowart describes that experience as being like "coming out of a fog." For the first time since his harrowing burn treatment ordeal, his sleep became normal and his depression lifted.

It was during this stay that I met Don Cowart and we began early discussions of a film that would eventually come to be known as *Dax's Case*. I still call him Don because that is how I know him, but he legally changed his name to Dax in the summer of 1982.

Some commentators on the film speculate that this change of name reflects some personal metamorphosis that Cowart went through during his lengthy rehabilitation period. But Cowart offers a simpler explanation. As a blind man with impaired hearing, he often found himself responding to comments addressed to others bearing the name of Don. I accepted his reasons for changing his name but asked him not to think the poorer of me for persisting in calling him Don.

It would be easy to believe that *Dax's Case,* more than five years in the making, served as a crucible for Don Cowart's rehabilitation. During this time, new hope and independence came into his life. He started a mail-order specialty foods business in Henderson using his creative powers. He moved into his own house. He became an articulate spokesperson for "the right to die" under auspices of Concern for Dying. And he married a former high school classmate in February 1983.

There is always another chapter, however. Even now, Don's life continues to shift. His first venture in business did not succeed financially. His second marriage ended unhappily. Amid failure has also come achievement. He returned to law school at Texas Tech University in Lubbock, where he completed his law degree in May and passed the bar in the summer of 1986. He set up a small law practice in Henderson and has recently taken in his first partner. He continues to represent his views on patient rights at educational symposiums and public forums. In time, he hopes to become a specialist in personal injury cases.

The film project was a crucible to Don Cowart in that it helped him reshape his life in dramatic ways. This retelling of the Cowart story has played a key role in his own reconstruction of a personal and public identity. His achievements in this regard have surpassed anything he, his family, or his physicians dared imagine. But this process of making a new life for himself is far from over. Only time will tell if *Dax's Case* is a heroic story with a happy or a tragic ending.

A Memoir: Dax's Case Twelve Years Later ⚕ *Robert B. White*

ON MAY 1, 1974, I CONSULTED WITH AN ATTORNEY regarding thorny legal and ethical questions raised by a young man who was both his client and my patient; the young man was demanding to die. Ten months previously he had suffered massive burns and he now insisted that life-sustaining treatment of those burns be stopped. Acceding to that request would mean his certain death.

On May 1, 1986, I received an invitation to attend the graduation ceremony at which this same man received the degree of doctor of jurisprudence. That man is Dax Cowart.

This coincidence of dates is only one of many extraordinary events in my relationship with Dax from its stormy beginning in 1974 to the triumph of the human spirit represented by his graduation from law school. At our first meeting it was immediately apparent that he was strong willed and determined, unbroken by months of unimaginable physical and emotional pain. His demand to die raised crucial medical, legal, ethical, and psychological issues. And the urgency of his clinical condition allowed no time for leisurely reflection or extended scholarly debate of the issues.

For the entirety of the twelve years since that meeting, Dax Cowart has disturbed my peace of mind, as I am sure he has disturbed all who have seen either *Dax's Case* or *Please Let Me Die.*[1] But it is fitting that my peace of mind be disturbed by the issues Dax raised, and I hope he has disturbed the peace of mind of all who have given thought to such matters.

The miracles of medical technology that allowed Dax Cowart to survive the extensive burns he suffered in July 1973, medical miracles from which he demanded release through death, have long since become outmoded. Since 1973 new technologies have appeared almost daily—advances that allow us often to maintain human life beyond the point of purpose, meaning, or hope. But during those years advances in legal and ethical thought have lagged far behind innovations in life-sustaining technology. In the aseptic, impersonal language of modern medicine, the heavy weapons in the physician's battle against his implacable adversary, death, are the "life-support systems." With these "systems" we physicians can now fend off death as never before. But with increasing frequency our triumphs over death force patients to plead for release from an existence they no longer wish to endure. Or our victories force their children or spouses to beg us to stop our fight and let death prevail. And at times our new-found power even forces family members to the unthinkable act of a mercy killing. At other times our technology presses life into an infant so tiny or malformed that it can never be whole or even truly human, infants whom nature never intended to survive the moment of birth. These advances prolong life in those of the elderly who are diapered and sequestered in nursing homes, as they babble away their final days—secured by ampules of antibiotics against pneumonia, the old man's friend, as it was known long ago.

But Dax was no infant incapable of speech or reason. He was not a demented old man. He was no Karen Quinlan, insensate in the darkness of brain death and sustained only by the regulated sigh of a respirator. He was no terminal cancer patient refusing a treatment which would at most postpone for only a little while a certain death. He was no deranged mental patient irrationally bent on self-destruction.

He was an intelligent, articulate, and well-educated young man who persistently demanded to die. He voiced this demand from the very first day of his injury in July 1973 when he was blinded and burned in the explosion of a propane gas transmission line near which by pure chance he and his father stood. His father died within hours; Dax survived.

At our first meeting ten months later, just a few days after Dax's admission to the third of the hospitals in which he had been confined continuously since his injury, he persisted in his request to be allowed to die. He refused to give permission for his surgeon to perform a desperately needed skin graft. He raged daily when lowered into the Hubbard tank to have his burns painfully bathed in an antiseptic solution of chlorox and water.

The question of whether he was mentally competent to refuse these lifesaving treatments posed a harsh dilemma for his surgeon who asked me to conduct a psychiatric evaluation. I found Dax Cowart to be mentally able to make a rational and informed decision either to accept or to refuse treatment. Although I was confident of my opinion, the circumstances were so unusual and the questions involved were so complex and troubling that I asked a trusted colleague to do an independent evaluation. My colleague also found Dax competent, and was as deeply troubled as I about the possible consequences of our opinion. Were we contributing to the death of a man who later might find value and meaning in life? Not a pleasant thought! With proper care this young man would undoubtedly survive; he might again find life worthwhile, even though blind, severely scarred, and maimed—with no fingers on his right hand and only a stub of a thumb on his scarred left. Other than giving an opinion that he was mentally competent, what else could a psychiatric consultant contribute to the care of a man who had suffered more than most could bear and who insisted he did not want life on the terms he faced? These terms demanded even more suffering in order to achieve the life of a blind cripple.

An active, vigorous, athletic man prior to his injury, Dax Cowart did not want life as a blind and maimed person, no longer able to ride in a rodeo, fly a jet plane, or do most of the things that he valued. But he could think, and his thoughts were clear and incisive. He used those thoughts to assert his autonomy and his will, hurling his demand to die at all who would listen. This racked his mother with despair and grief, though she bore it all with quiet dignity. It deviled his surgeon. It perplexed psychiatric consultants. It disconcerted attorneys.

In addition to giving emotional support, I was able to help Dax by altering his pain medication (done in collaboration with a colleague from anesthesiology), and by assisting him with his request that his attorney take his case to court to determine whether his demand to die could be legally enforced. I also supported his mother as well as I could, and suggested that she withdraw from the frequent arguments she was having with her son about his wish to die; these always ended in a painful impasse and settled nothing.

What a troubling and perplexing case! I had never confronted such before (nor have I since, for that matter)—nor had any of my colleagues with whom I discussed the matter. During each visit to Dax's bedside a thought intruded uncontrollably into my mind: if I were Dax, I too would choose to die. But such personal views can be a treacherous guide to medical care. It is the same guide that leads many physicians to insist that they are obligated to sustain life at all cost, no matter the circumstance or the consequence.

Another observation troubled me. In his pain and helpless frustration Dax had episodic rages in which he flailed his maimed arms in helpless fury as he screamed at his mother that he wanted to die. Was his demand to die a protest against the helpless and infantile state into which he had been forced for so many months, a state in which he was totally at the mercy of those who cared for him? Of course, no one intentionally imposed such helplessness on him; it was inherent and unavoidable in the treatment of his grave injuries.

His rages had qualities of a childlike tantrum, and it was toward his mother and his physician that his fury was primarily directed. It was on them that he also felt most dependent. Like an infant, for months he had to be fed, bathed, toileted, and moved about (even to change position in his bed). He could not see; his stumplike hands had no fingers or nerves with which to feel. Every vestige of adult independence had been destroyed except for his mind and his words. His mind and his words were powerful, and he used them very effectively to assert his autonomy and impose his will. How better to assert his autonomy than to shout at his doctor and his mother, "Let me die."

Dax's Case poignantly conveys the impact of this upon his surgeon, Dr. Duane Larson. It ran counter to every value and every fiber of Dr. Larson's identity as a competent and dedicated physician. How could he agree? And certainly Dax's mother was equally compelled to argue against her son's demands. And they argued about this almost every day, usually heatedly. So as a consultant I pondered this possibility: Was Dax's demand to die predominantly an effort to assert his autonomy and independence or was it truly the expression of a deeply held wish to die? Certainly no other demand could have exerted such a profound impact on the two people on whom he was most dependent at that point—his surgeon and his mother.

As a psychiatric consultant to the burn unit at my hospital, I had for years observed that severely burned patients inevitably regress to some degree of childlike behavior, as all people do when helpless, in great pain, and totally dependent on others for long periods of time. As a psychoanalyst, I knew well that behavior can communicate various levels of meaning and that sometimes the most readily apparent meaning of a communication may not be the most important meaning. Often the important message may be disguised and difficult to discern and quite different from the apparent meaning. Moreover, there was the complex issue of ambivalence in human behavior, that is, people often are quite divided in their intent. They may very much want a certain goal and simultaneously not want it. So the surface message, "I want to die," might not be the whole story. In fact, I had to concern myself with the possibility that it was not even the main story.

Could an important clue lie in those very moments when Dax

regressed to childlike behavior? When a small child is hurt and helpless he or she predictably will turn hurt into anger toward the parents and others who provide care and on whom he or she depends. The child feels that if the parent (or other caretakers) really cared they would not inflict such pain. The child can only conclude that the distress is their doing, that they caused the hurt deliberately, and then understandably becomes angry with them. It appeared to me that Dax, in his regressed moments, turned upon his caretakers in a similar manner. His mother caught the brunt of his rages, but his physician also received his full share as Dax frustrated Dr. Larson in his efforts to save his patient's life.

But I do not insist that these thoughts about Dax's motivations are correct. The main point I wish to emphasize by including them in my reflections is that the simple, straightforward, "I want to die," may not have been the whole story. It could have been a grave error to assume that it was. To accede immediately to Dax's wish to die could have been disastrous. On the other hand, it would have been an equally grave error to discount his demand to die as nothing more than some transient psychological aberration or symptom of a serious mental illness.

I think we shall never know whether Dax wholeheartedly wanted to die. But he demanded to die, and that was the issue that had to be dealt with at the time. All that I can say in retrospect is that shortly after I supported his wish to have the question settled by a court, he consented to treatment and, to the relief of all concerned, he did not raise the issue again. So Dax did not die, but through the years he has continued to press his view that he had the right to die in May 1974.

We must find a judicious and reasoned response to this view that Dax stoutly maintains to this day. Our response must be one that safeguards patients when such requests are a symptom of mental illness. It must protect patients who act impulsively as a result of temporary exhaustion and stress. Surgeons who treat severely burned patients know well that patients sometimes despair and ask that the treatment be stopped, only later to agree that their request should not have been met. Patients must also be safeguarded against unscrupulous physicians or family members who, out of hope for personal gain, request that a patient be allowed to die. Perhaps most of all, patients must be protected against those physicians who out of personal bias blindly adhere to the view that human life must be sustained as long as possible and regardless of the wishes of the patient. Above all, we must safeguard the right of patients to decide their own fate—including those who are too incapacitated to state their wishes during their illness but who made their desires clearly known in writing at an earlier time, as with a living will. Likewise, we must honor the right of self-determination for those who make their wishes known in a creditably witnessed verbal statement, as in the case of Brother Joseph Fox, the New York priest who, through court order in 1979, was kept alive by a respirator despite his emphatic wish to the contrary, a wish which he had made known before he became comatose.[2]

And finally, I believe that the time has come for physicians, attorneys, and judges to face squarely the question of euthanasia. Ironically, the very procedures and machines which increase our victories over disease now press us to provide a merciful end for those patients who resolutely request release from a struggle against death when that struggle becomes no longer bearable.

But what policies should guide the physician in making a responsible decision regarding a patient's request to die? No longer is this a purely academic issue of interest primarily only to the ethicists and philosophers. Increasingly, thoughtful clinicians and people generally are saying: "Enough of your oath, Hippocrates; I demand the right to choose death over life when disease makes that life unbearable." Few have pointed the way in this direction more courageously than Sigmund Freud and his compassionate personal physician, Max Schur.[3]

In the final days of his long bout with cancer of the mouth, Freud, then eighty-three years of age, clearly stated his wish for release from meaningless suffering when he told his doctor the following: "My Dear Schur, you remember our first talk. You promised me that you would help me when I could no longer carry on. It is only torture now and has no longer any sense."

In that first talk to which Freud refers, a talk held over ten years previously, Schur had promised his patient that he would shield him from pain whenever Freud requested. So, responding to Freud's wish, Schur injected a large dose of morphine—a dose of 20 mg. Frail, elderly, and decimated by disease, Freud had never before received narcotics in his long siege with cancer; consequently, he had developed no tolerance for the opiates. Soon after the injection he quietly went to sleep, and did not awaken again, his final rest assured by a second dose some hours after the first.

What a gift! What a priceless gift. What a fine and noble example of the dedicated physician who provides his patient with the best of care. What a contrast to "life-support systems" and to physicians and hospital administrators who seek judicial decrees to protect them legally should they dare provide a patient with such humane care as that given by Dr. Schur. What a contrast to those attorneys and judges who feel that a patient's request to die should be granted only through the clash of adversarial procedure such as that which so long denied the priest, Brother Fox, his emphatic request never to be kept alive by a respirator. What a contrast to the court decree which forced the mentally retarded Joseph Saikewicz to be subjected to a futile course of painful chemotherapy in order that his leukemia might be kept at bay for a few more tortured months;[4] or to the decree concerning the cancer-ridden John Storar whose suffering was prolonged despite the strong objection of his aged mother.[5] John Storar was profoundly mentally retarded and had spent his entire life institutionalized.

Of course, it is not possible to place Schur's courageous decision into the hands of every physician unless we also provide safeguards against abuse. The possibilities for misuse are too great. But surely some method can be found to provide accountability and adequate safeguards against abuse without unduly cumbersome and time-consuming judicial procedures. If a patient can give a physician permission (properly recorded in the hospital medical record) to perform very risky experimental surgery that provides very little chance of recovery, say the installation of a mechanical heart, should not that same patient also have the right to grant his or her physician a properly documented permission to end a life made unbearable by disease?

These are the thoughts prompted by your case, Dax Cowart. You have troubled my mind greatly but, again, let me say how indebted I am to you for troubling me so. You made me think about unthinkable problems. In your new career in the law I hope that you now can help to untangle the complex, cumbersome rulings and court decisions which would have completely obstructed Dr. Schur from performing his wonderful act of mercy in his care of Sigmund Freud. Such court decrees obstructed humane and reasoned medical care in the case of the old priest, Joseph Fox, and the two helpless, mentally retarded men, John Storar and Joseph Saikewicz. And I am sure there are countless others. I may someday be among that countless number—as you again may also be. We must hurry, Dax Cowart; the task is long; the time is short.

NOTES

1. *Dax's Case.* An hour-long documentary film produced by Unicorn Media, Inc., for Concern for Dying, Inc., New York, 1985. *Please Let Me Die: The Wish of a Blind Severely Maimed Burn Patient.* A thirty-minute videotape produced by Robert B. White, M.D., through the facilities of the Department of Educational Television, University of Texas Medical Branch, Galveston, 1974.

2. G. J. Annas, "Quinlan, Saikewicz and Now Brother Fox," *Hastings Center Report* 10 (June 1980): 20–21; G. J. Annas, "Help from the Dead: The Cases of Brother Fox and John Storar," *Hastings Center Report* 11 (June 1981): 19–20; J. J. Paris, "Court Intervention and the Diminution of Patients' Rights: The Case of Brother Joseph Fox," *New England Journal of Medicine* 303 (1980): 876–78; J. J. Paris, "The Conclusion of the Brother Fox Case," *New England Journal of Medicine* 304 (1981): 1424–25.

3. Max Schur, *Freud: Living and Dying* (New York: International University Press, 1972).

4. Annas, "Quinlan," 20–21; G. J. Annas, "The Incompetent's Right to Die: The Case of Joseph Saikewicz," *Hastings Center Report* 8 (February 1978): 21–23. Saikewicz, a sixty-seven-year-old man with the IQ of a two year old, had been institutionalized all his life. He died in 1976 while his case requiring treatment for acute myeloblastic monocetic leukemia was under appeal. The Massachusetts Supreme Judicial Court later affirmed a lower court decision to withhold treatment.

5. Annas, "Help from the Dead," 19–20. John Storar, an institutionalized fifty-two-year-old man with a mental age of eighteen months, was given court-ordered blood transfusions to counteract terminal bladder cancer despite his widowed mother's express wish to let him die.

"Who Is a Doctor to Decide Whether a Person Lives or Dies?" Reflections on Dax's Case

James F. Childress, Courtney C. Campbell

THE FACT THAT DAX COWART IS ALIVE TODAY, HAV-ing finished law school and living a productive life, may be viewed as a triumph and vindication of medical paternalism over patient autonomy. After all, Cowart, who suffered severe burns as a result of an accidental explosion of natural gas in 1973, was given medical treatment for his own benefit despite his numerous refusals and repeated requests to die. Dax's case has become so prominent in biomedical ethics because it poses such an important and dramatic conflict between moral duties to benefit patients and to respect their wishes. The original videotape, *Please Let Me Die*, which presents Dr. Robert White's psychiatric interview with Dax Cowart, effectively challenges viewers to consider how they would balance the principles of respect for persons and patient benefit when a patient refuses life-prolonging treatment even though he or she is not terminally ill, i.e., is not irreversibly and imminently dying, and life could be prolonged indefinitely with reasonably good quality.

In our use of this videotape in courses, the most common response is that Dax should have been allowed to exercise his moral and legal right to choose death. Viewers are convinced by what they see and hear—Dax Cowart's powerful and lucid voice emerging from his badly burned, scarred, and pain-racked body to assert his right to make his own choices and to ask, "Who is a doctor to decide whether a person lives or dies?" Of course, they always want to know the outcome—what happened to the patient? And they are often stunned by the report that Dax Cowart subsequently accepted treatment and is doing very well. This report forces them to reconsider their original judgment that he should have been allowed to die. We find that this case illuminates several issues in the debate about medical paternalism and patient autonomy. It does not serve merely as an illustration of a preset balance of patient benefit and patient autonomy; its very complexities force qualifications, or at the very least, clarifications of theories of paternalism. [1]

THE NATURE OF MEDICAL PATERNALISM

It can be assumed that the end of medicine and health care is patient benefit. Even if the traditional first duty of physicians and other health care professionals is *primum non nocere*—first of all or at least do no harm—there would be no point to medicine and health care if professionals did not aim at patient benefit, including cure, prolongation of life, and relief of pain and suffering. However, recognition that the end of medicine is patient benefit does not take us very far. Patient benefit obviously includes many different specific ends, and those ends usually cannot be obtained without means that have risks, burdens, and costs. Hence, even if patient benefit cannot be defined apart from medical competence, it also cannot be defined apart from a framework of values that can identify some outcomes as benefits and others as harms or burdens and assign weights to different positive and negative outcomes.

But if judgments about patient benefit necessarily presuppose values, then the question immediately emerges: Whose values should be determinative? In Dax's case, we might ask whether his values or the values of his mother, the physicians and other health care professionals involved in his care, or others should determine actions. It is an oversimplification to pose the conflict as one between beneficence and autonomy, because it is also in part a conflict about

24

whose interpretation of beneficence will triumph. As Dax Cowart has noted, physicians often try "to benefit the patient on their own terms rather than the patient's. My case was an example of where the two are not the same." [2] Nevertheless, because the claim of medical authority to override the patient's wishes rests on the professional's commitment and competence to benefit the patient, and the claim of the patient rests on the right of self-determination, we will state the conflict in terms of beneficence and respect for persons, with respect for autonomy as a subset of the principle of respect for persons. Paternalism may be defined as nonacquiescence to a person's wishes, choices, or actions for that person's own benefit. In general it assigns primacy to beneficence over respect for persons including their autonomy.

According to the principle of respect for persons, autonomous patients should have the right to make their own choices to accept or to refuse medical treatments, including lifesaving medical treatments, as long as their choices do not impose serious harms or burdens on others. To deny or override this right is disrespectful because it insults the autonomous patient by imposing on him or her someone else's conception of patient benefit and of the good life and death. Nietzsche once suggested that all assistance is an insult, but it is more defensible to hold that all assistance against an autonomous person's informed and voluntary refusal is an insult. A basic objection to appeals to the principle of respect for persons, rooted in the Kantian and Millian traditions, is their failure to attend to time and to community. We want to show that the principle of respect for persons can and should be interpreted to allow for time and community, but in ways that will not justify treating an autonomous patient against his or her informed and voluntary choices where those choices do not impose serious risks or burdens on others.

Our formulation of what the principle of respect for persons implies for autonomous patient choices is subject to both internal and external limits, some of which are expressed in the following chart:

| | Adverse Effects | | |
		On Self	On Others
Patient's	Autonomous	1	2
Choices	Nonautonomous	3	4

Even the autonomous patient's choices are constrained by several *external* limits, some of which can be morally justified. Such limits include societal and institutional policies of allocating resources, regulations on the use of drugs, professional standards of care, and the professional's conscience. Many of these limits and others restrict a patient's right to choose treatments, rather than his or her right to refuse treatments. But even the negative right to refuse treatments may be justifiably limited when those actions seriously harm others. Thus, when serious adverse effects of a patient's choices fall on others (2 and 4 in the above chart), the patient's choices may sometimes be justifiably restricted. However, one external limit that clinicians often recognize—the family's wishes—is morally unwarranted in the care of autonomous patients apart from the few imaginable cases where the patient's refusal of lifesaving treatment would subject the family to serious harms or burdens.

In addition, there are *internal* limits. If a patient cannot make autonomous choices (see 3 on the chart), it is not insulting or disrespectful to override his or her choices. And the clinician's duty to benefit and not to harm the patient requires actions to protect the patient from his or her nonautonomous choices.

These points can be explicated by reference to *Dax's Case.* Most actions against a patient's wishes involve efforts to protect both the patient and others; hence they are rarely purely paternalistic. Impure paternalistic actions aim at the patient's welfare but also at the welfare of others. In Dax's case, the clinicians identified his welfare as the primary reason for their refusal to acquiesce in his expressed wish to die, but they also invoked harms and burdens to others. For example, Dr. White expressed concern about the "unfair burden" that would be imposed on Cowart's mother if treatment were discontinued. Rex Houston worried about the negative effect of Dax's death on the lawsuit against the company that maintained the pipeline that had leaked the gas; Dax's death could reduce the amount of the settlement for the family. And some clinicians, such as Dr. Duane Larson, felt that Dax's refusal placed them in a situation where their own moral values would be compromised. The more paternalism is "impure" and the foreseen harms or burdens to others are real, rather than mere rationalizations, the more defensible the intervention is.

Paternalism may involve active or passive nonacquiesence in the patient's choices. In *active* nonacquiescence, the paternalist refuses to accept a patient's request for nonintervention or noninterference, while in *passive* nonacquiescence, a paternalist refuses to carry out the wishes or choices of a patient or to assist the patient in his or her action. It is easier, *ceteris paribus*, to justify passive paternalism than active paternalism, in part because passive paternalism reflects the professional's autonomy, which means that he or she is not a mere instrument or tool of the patient's wishes, and in part because passive paternalism leaves the patient other options.

In *Dax's Case,* the professionals were actively paternalistic when they refused to honor his request for ninintervention and discontinuation of treatment. Yet some of their arguments were more complex. For example, Dax's request was not honored, because to some practitioners it implied a "willingness to participate in his suicide" (White) or because "to not treat this patient is in a sense to kill him" (Larson). Of course, their objections to participating in Dax's suicide or killing him may have rested on their interpretation of societal rules against assisting suicide and mercy killing, as well as on their judgments about his welfare. However, questions could be raised about their interpretation of these rules.

Finally, paternalism may be *hard* or *soft*, depending on the role the patient's own values play in the decision-making process. This distinction focuses on the *source* of the values that are invoked to justify paternalism. In *Dax's Case,* his clinicians, his mother, and other relevant parties such as the family attorney often displayed hard paternalism in their appeal to values (such as religious salvation) and rankings of values (such as the priority of life over quality of life) that were alien to Dax himself. Hard paternalism is usually more dificult to justify because it discounts the patient's own values in favor of someone else's values, often presented as "objective" values. Interestingly, when Dax's *own* values—particularly the values of freedom and self-determination—were invoked as the reason for not acquiescing in his choice, he decided to accept further surgery (e.g., Larson's challenge to Dax in *Dax's Case*). Soft paternalism, which takes the patient's own values seriously, even against his or her expressed wishes, is more defensible, *ceteris paribus*, than hard paternalism, which imposes alien values.

Because of the principle of respect for persons, there is a strong moral presumption against paternalistic actions by physicians and other health care professionals. However, such paternalistic actions can be justified under some circumstances. The pattern of justification that seems acceptable combines beneficence and respect for persons; it may be characterized as a principle of *limited beneficence*. It builds on professional beneficence toward the patient but limits and constrains that beneficence by respect for the patient's autonomous wishes, choices, and actions. According to one suggestive image, beneficence provides the engine—the motivation and direction—of medical care, while the patient's wishes, choices, and actions determine the tracks along which it runs.

In order to justify paternalistic interventions without violating the principle of respect for persons, it is necessary, first of all, to rebut the presumption of an adult patient's competence to make his or her own choices. Second, it is necessary to show that the patient would suffer serious harm without actions on his or her behalf. The third condition for justified paternalism is proportionality: The intervention cannot be morally justified unless it would probably be effective and its positive results would probably outweigh its negative results. Fourth, even when paternalistic interventions are justified, the least restrictive, least humiliating, and least insulting means should be employed. In general, the more *impure* the paternalistic action is (that is, the more it prevents harms to parties other than the patient), the *softer* it is (that is, the more it appeals to the patient's own values), and the more its nonacquiescence is *passive* rather than active, the more easily it can be justified. (The above conditions for justification apply mainly to active paternalism.)

According to this analysis, paternalism takes many different forms, not all of which are equally objectionable. In particular, limited active paternalism, which applies beneficence within the limits of respect for persons, can be defended, when the above conditions are met. However, most commentators agree that the first necessary conditions of that model were not met in Dax's case, at least at the time of the interview with Dr. White (ten months after the accident), for Dax was an autonomous decision maker. If this interpretation is accurate, then active paternalistic interventions would not have been limited by the principle of respect for persons and would have been unjustified. However, a closer analysis shows the complexity of this case as well as the difficulty of interpreting the limits set by the principle of respect for persons, particularly in determining whether people are making autonomous choices and what their choices really are. Our analysis of these complexities will consider both time and community, which, according to critics, are neglected by proponents of the principles of respect for persons and limited paternalism.

THE AMBIGUITY OF AUTONOMY

The principle of respect for persons entails respect for their autonomous wishes, choices, and actions. However, as noted earlier, this principle is subject to both internal and external limits. Questions about internal limits emerged in several ways in Dax's case.

As Bruce Miller has suggested, it is important to distinguish two senses of autonomy: effective deliberation and freedom of action. When Cowart began to refuse treatment, the attending physicians raised questions about his autonomy. Focusing on "effective deliberation," Dr. Charles Baxter maintained that in the "shock phase," burn survivors are "incompetent" to make decisions about their treatment. Dax's mother concurred in this assessment, concluding that "his condition was so bad that he could not make judgments about what to do with the rest of his life, and whether or not to have treatment."

By contrast, Sharon Imbus and Bruce Zawacki, members of the burn team for the Los Angeles County–USC Medical Center, hold that "during the first few hours of hospitalization . . . even the most severely burned patient is usually alert and mentally competent."[3] Thus, their burn team takes "an *aggressive* approach to decision making to preserve patient autonomy," giving patients sufficient information about their condition and prospects and asking them whether they wish to choose between full therapy and ordinary care. They contend that such patients both exercise more "self-determination" and receive more "empathy" and that the mortality rates have not increased in the burn unit. They do not extend this aggressive approach to autonomy to all burn patients, but only to those for whom survival is unprecedented.

Critics of this approach contend that even in the early period the severely burned patient suffers from such physical and emotional shock that he or she cannot participate in decision making and, furthermore, that early maximal treatment is warranted because of uncertainties about which patients can be salvaged, particularly as treatments improve. Thus, critics contend that, at least in the early period, the first two conditions for justified paternalism are met in the case of severely burned patients. Such patients are not competent to decide because of physical and emotional shock, and, because physicians cannot be certain about which patients can be salvaged, they should provide maximal treatment to all, for withholding treatment at that point guarantees death.

Dax Cowart refused treatment from the time of the accident. He first asked a farmer who approached to get him a gun so that he could end his life; he then asked the rescue squad not to take him to the hospital and the physicians in the emergency room not to treat him. Interventions against his wishes at those points were justified in order to gain time to be able to determine his competence and to make an accurate diagnosis and prognosis, which could not be made immediately. Only when these conditions were met could his choices have been autonomous in the sense of effective deliberation with adequate information resulting in voluntary choices. Dax also indicates that he had nightmares and hallucinations during one period—believing, for example, that the staff was using him as a guinea pig for their experiments—but that by the time of the interview with Dr. White he could look back with what he describes as "a clear mind" and admit that it didn't happen. Choices made under those earlier conditions would not have been autonomous.

However, at some point during the next ten months, he became autonomous in this sense. Most commentators and viewers of *Please Let Me Die* agree that by the time of this interview Dax Cowart was autonomous in the sense of effective deliberation. Indeed, the efforts of the physicians to have him declared incompetent, so that they could continue corrective surgery as well as other treatments, were rebuffed by the psychiatric reports. Still one question is when during the ten months he became competent and had adequate information to make his own decisions about treatment/nontreatment.

The second sense of autonomy—freedom of action—raises some interesting questions. Are persons who display effective deliberation to be considered autonomous when, as in Dax's case, they are physically unable to act freely on their choices? If we hold that the principle of respect for persons engenders obligations to acquiesce in the wishes, choices, and actions of patients, it is reasonable to ask what this principle requires when a patient's deliberative choices cannot be realized in actions.

In considering whether Cowart was autonomous, most commentators have found that he passed the threshold for autonomy because of his capacity for effective deliberation, along with the authenticity of his choices, that is, their consistency with and reflection of values that he had affirmed throughout his life. Yet it is important not to neglect the problems raised by the fact that he was incapable of autonomy as freedom of action because he was physically unable to act on his wishes and choices. (We will return to authenticity later). For example, Dax indicated that he did not "intend to die from the infection" that would result from the discontinuation of the daily tankings. However, his unwillingness to die this way meant that to die required the assistance of others. Dr. White insists that, "in essence, he was asking others to participate in his suicide." Hence, the refusal of physicians and other health care professionals to act on his wishes may have stemmed in part from their refusal to be mere instruments of the chosen ends of a patient, particularly in violation of professional codes and criminal laws that prohibit assisted suicide. If he had planned to rely on his family or friends for assistance, they would have faced similar questions.

It is also important to distinguish, as Robert Nozick suggests, autonomy as a "side-constraint" from autonomy as an "end-state." As a side-constraint, autonomy limits what we may do to and for others even to benefit them. Autonomy in this sense determines the channels along which benefits flow to patients from medical actions; it limits paternalistic interventions. However, because Dax Cowart was not autonomous in the sense of *free action,* in contrast to effective deliberation, it might be argued that continuation of treatment was essential to restore his autonomy as free action. In such an argument autonomy is understood not as a side-constraint but as an end-state to be realized through the continuation of therapeutic procedures. This understanding of autonomy as the end-state of free action appears in Dr. Larson's recollection of what he told Cowart: "If you want to die, at least let me fix those hands, at least you can do something with them. Then if you want to commit suicide, that's for you to decide."

It is tempting to construe this pursuit of the end-state of autonomy as nonpaternalistic, but viewing autonomy as a benefit to be sought simply expands the traditional understanding of medical benefits, and allowing it to override autonomy as a side-constraint still fits the paternalistic model. There are good reasons to be suspicious of this effort to recast the problem in order to avoid an apparent conflict with the principle of respect for persons. Nevertheless, our analysis is intended to identify the ambiguous nature of autonomy—and appeals to autonomy—in decisions about treatment and nontreatment in Dax's case as well as other such cases. How the professional responds may depend on which feature of autonomy— effective deliberation or free action—is emphasized, and on whether autonomy is conceived as a side-constraint or as an end-state.

THE TEMPORAL DIMENSION:
DISCERNING PATIENT PREFERENCES OVER TIME

Dax Cowart's initial requests to die were "literally ignored" because of a judgment that the physical and emotional "shock" of the accident and burns had rendered him incompetent to engage in effective deliberation. Often in emergency situations or life-threatening refusals, temporary interventions and treatments are necessary and morally justified in order to gain time to discern with greater accuracy the patient's wishes and choices. Even John Stuart Mill's classic essay *On Liberty* justified a temporary intervention to make sure that a person about to cross a dangerous bridge was acting autonomously—that is, was competent, understood the risks, and chose voluntarily to cross the bridge. The temporal dimension is very important in an analysis of Dax's case, and such an analysis may suggest further complexities because of the different parties' views of how *time* could play a role in confirming, ratifying, or altering Dax's wishes and choices and their own responses.

Too often crisis-oriented medicine and ethical analysis arbitrarily cut off the present from the past and the future, even though the self exists in time and develops over time. Thus, one important index of autonomy is what has been termed *authenticity*, particularly the consistency of a person's wishes, choices, and actions with the values he or she has represented or expressed over time. The intuitive idea of authenticity is "acting in character," and we wonder whether choices or actions are autonomous if they are "out of character" with what we know of the person over time. If they are "in character," we are less likely to suspect that they do not represent genuine autonomy.

33

This idea of authenticity has been a principal and pervasive feature in Cowart's interpretation and defense of his refusal of life-sustaining treatments. His desire to die was formed by values that had shaped his life in the past, especially his conception of the good life as the free, independent, and active life, which, for him, included sports, rodeo, flying, etc. "He always wanted to do things for himself and in his own way." Thus, Dax's refusal of life-sustaining treatment was an "authentic" choice when measured against the values he had consistently affirmed, both prior to and after his accident.

By contrast, the burn therapist, Dr. Larson, appealed to the temporal dimension to suggest that Dax's request was inauthentic and out of character: "If you're the *kind of person* I've been led to believe you were *before* you were burned, then don't ask us to let you die, because that means we're killing you." Although this move from "letting die" to "killing" is highly problematic in the circumstances, the main point is to appeal to Dax's values over time in order to justify continuing treatment. Significantly, it was this self-described "attack" by Larson that resulted in Cowart's decision to drop his objections to further therapeutic surgery on his hands.

Dax's refusal up to that time had been based on a further temporal dimension of the case—his vision of the future. Although Dax had repeatedly requested to be allowed to die, Dr. Robert Meier reports that his serious refusal of treatment began after an "off-handed remark" by a surgical resident that the therapy, and consequent pain, could involve a "number of years." By contrast, for Larson, the most important aspect of time in Dax's case was the time already "invested." Cowart had already invested twelve months in a most excruciating ordeal, and to give up then would be like a marathon runner quitting with one mile to go. It is unclear whether Larson's opinion would have changed significantly if less time had been invested.

Often paternalistic actions are initiated or continued, even if presently resisted, on the basis of an appeal to the patient's future consent or subsequent ratification, similar to what parents express when they say to their children—"You'll thank me for this later."

Dax attributes this belief to the physicians and nurses who tried to keep him alive: "I also feel that they probably were under the impression that in the end I would be glad that they did and that I would be grateful in the long run that they did force me to undergo this treatment."[4] Ada Cowart, Dax's mother, believes that *time* has indeed ratified her decision to continue treatment against her son's wishes: "Looking back over the last ten years, I think I made the right decision. . . . Now that he's married, enjoying life and his business, I know it's right now."

Dax himself has refused to offer retrospective ratification of the decisions on his behalf but against his wishes. And this refusal makes his case even more interesting than it might have been otherwise. This refusal to say "thank you for saving my life" troubles many physicians and other health care professionals, even those not involved in his care. For example, in a Medical Center Hour at the University of Virginia in March 1984, Dax presented his case, contending that he had been treated wrongly even though he was now glad to be alive and had achieved a quality of life that he had not anticipated at the time of his accident and during the course of his treatments. Several questions from the audience focused on what was perceived to be his inconsistency in being glad to be alive while being ungrateful to professionals for their efforts to keep him alive against his wishes. But, in his view, the decision to continue treatment against his autonomous wishes was morally unjustifiable paternalism then and now, because "the ends do not justify the means." It was a form of disrespect to him as a person.

This discrepancy in perspectives indicates that it is insufficient to appeal to future ratification as a basis for continuing treatment against a patient's wishes in the present. In this case, the person who was most affected by the decision has never ratified it. And it is quite conceivable that things could have been very different—for example, Dax did attempt to commit suicide at least twice because of various difficulties. Furthermore, even though he is pleased with the outcome, that is, where he is today, Dax contends that even if he could have foreseen that enjoyable outcome he would still have refused treatment because of the pain and suffering it involved. And he would make the same decision under the same circumstances again, but, he concedes, he "might not make the decision [to refuse treatment] as readily."[5] (Incidentally, he justified his name change from Donald to Dax because Dax was easier for him to hear, but it may also serve another function: It marks a sharp break in his identification of himself over time and a separation of the present and the future from the painful past.)

An appeal to future ratification is insufficient to justify paternalistic interventions, and it is also unnecessary to justify such actions. Such appeals at the time of decision making simply reflect the agent's hope; they are unnecessary for justification. To make justification hinge on *actual* ratification is inappropriate because many patients never gain or regain the capacity to ratify others' decisions and actions on their behalf. And *predicted* ratification is redundant and restrictive. It is redundant because the prediction is based on the other criteria identified earlier for justified paternalism; it is restrictive because some paternalistic interventions may be justified even when it cannot be predicted with confidence that the patient will ever ratify them. For example, we believe that temporary paternalistic interventions were justified in order to gain time to determine and restore Dax's competence and to determine his prognosis as well as to discern his true wishes in the face of adequate information. Even though Dax now appears to ratify some of those decisions, but not others, their justification does not depend on his actual or his predicted ratification.

We have already suggested that paternalistic interventions are sometimes important to "gain time." Dr. White suggested that Dax "wait and see." And Mrs. Cowart believed it was important to "gain time" for other reasons as well. She wanted her son's treatment continued so that he could "realize his responsibility to God and to realize what he should be doing." Furthermore, she expressed concern that her son might subsequently change his mind and accept or even request treatment, but that his change of mind might come too late and "there would be nothing anyone could do to help him" if his early refusal was honored. In considering refusals of lifesaving treatments, it is important to allow for the possibility of changes over time in the wishes and choices of patients; hence, irreversible actions must be taken with the utmost caution. But mere possibilities should not be allowed to outweigh the reality of present autonomous dissent in determining whether treatment should be continued.

Past consent now repudiated by refusal may raise questions about the authenticity of the patient's choice, particularly if the past consent made sense in terms of the patient's long-term values. The idea of authenticity captures our sense that selves develop over time with persistent and enduring patterns and are not mere collections of choices and actions. And yet it would be a mistake to view authenticity as a criterion of autonomy. At most, considerations of authenticity should alert us to ask further questions. If the choice or action, such as refusal of life-sustaining treatment, is inconsistent with what we know of a person and his or her character, then we should seek justifications or explanations.

It is not only difficult to respect persons as persons because they change over time but also because they give conflicting signals at the same time. Often their wishes, choices, and actions are ambiguous. Then it is necessary to determine which wishes, choices, and actions to respect. It is difficult to determine at this point how clear-cut Dax's directives were at different times during the treatment. For example, in 1984 Dax indicated that his lawyer was probably right when he indicated that Dax had "wanted to live long enough to get the settlement from the oil company that we had sued in an action of negligence" regarding the maintenance of the pipeline that had exploded.[6] The suit was worth more while Dax was alive, and he wanted his family to be taken care of. However, once the suit was settled this concern ceased to be relevant, and most reports of the case acknowledge Dax's firm and persistent rejection of treatment.

Nevertheless, it is sometimes possible to point to a person's signals other than his or her explicit statements. The process of communication is very complex and requires attention to various verbal and nonverbal signs, as well as time for interaction. Attention to those other signs may tempt health care professionals and others who want to save the patient to believe that they have discerned the patient's "real" will to live, rather than to die. It is also tempting to read some other message into the patient's expressed wish to die. Although claims about the patient's real wishes or messages are not always mistaken, they need to be taken with caution when they are at odds with the patient's expressed wish to die. Because Dax finally submitted to treatment when he had apparently gained his victory, in part as a way to extricate himself from the system, it might be supposed that he had not really wanted to die and that his request to die was actually an attempt to expiate his feelings of guilt over his father's death, or a protest against fate, against the loss of control over his destiny, against his dependence and his being "at the mercy" of others, against inadequate attention to his pain and suffering, or against what he perceived as depersonalized and even incompetent care. At the very least, he wanted increased *control* over his life. Rights enable patients to become agents and, within limits, to direct their care. And, Dax emphasizes, he wanted the right to control, i.e., to make his own decisions, and to die.[7]

We believe that it was imperative to acknowledge Dax's right to decide for himself whether to accept or refuse treatment after enough time had elapsed to determine his prognosis, his competence, and his settled wishes. At some point paternalistic interventions were unjustified. Such interventions can be justified against the wishes of nonautonomous patients on grounds of both beneficence and respect for persons. But when the patient is sufficiently autonomous, respect for persons requires that the patient be allowed to make his or her own determinations of benefits. Nevertheless, familial or professional beneficence does not evaporate under pressure from patient autonomy. Respect for persons unleavened by care can appear as indifference to the life and death of others.

RESPECT FOR PERSONS IN THEIR COMMUNITIES

Appeals to the principle of respect for persons are often viewed with suspicion not only because they appear to remove people from time but also because they appear to remove people from communities. The original presentation of Dax's case in the videotape *Please Let Me Die* has been criticized because of the absence of the family, as well as other significant parties; *Dax's Case* adds these other characters. Certainly it is important to consider the social context of any patient's request to be allowed to die. People are not as distinct and as separate as some interpretations of the principle of respect for persons appear to suggest. This point not only suggests that "no man is an island" because actions have so many effects on others; it also implies that an individual's wishes often reflect the social context in ways that are sometimes overlooked.

Robert Burt argues that if we ignore "the emotional context" of Dax's invocation of the right to die, "we would find ourselves purporting to obey the wishes of a caricature," for his dependence led him to inquire about the wishes of others, not only to express his own wishes. His plea to be allowed to die, Burt notes, was perhaps "more a question to others about their wishes toward him" because he could not die, at least as he wanted to, without their active collaboration. Hence it is morally important for all parties to express, and for the patient to perceive, care. Such care by professionals, family members, and friends may require altering features of the patient's environment, for example, by reducing pain and gesturing concern. Without this social context of care, acquiescence in the patient's wishes may be (rightly) perceived as indifference rather than respect.

Expression of community through gestures of care and concern is an important but often neglected aspect of ethical policies, practices, and actions. For example, what do a relative's or a professional's actions symbolize about the patient's place in and significance for the community? Our chart above included some attention to the community, but mainly through the impact of a person's actions on others, and we argued that it is easier to justify overriding a person's wishes, choices, or actions when they have adverse effects on others than when those adverse effects fall only on the patient. But protecting the community, including individuals within the community, is not the same as expressing community. Dax recognizes that the people who wanted to keep him alive "had an honest concern for [his] well-being."[8] In short, they included him in their community. But such an expression of community, whether by the family or by health care professionals, may emphasize care or beneficence at the expense of respect. After unwarranted neglect because of fascination with individual autonomy, community is now rightly receiving a great deal of attention in biomedical ethics. But the turn toward community, as important and essential as it is, may become tyrannical if it is not limited by respect for persons.

It is easy to affirm community, but such affirmations should only be made in the spirit of realism. First, realism recognizes that community is often an ideal rather than a reality. Even if we are not strangers, we may not constitute a genuine community of shared values or we may not have enough knowledge of each other to know whether we constitute such a community. In the absence of community, rights are important to protect individual self-determination. Second, realism is needed not only because community is often only an ideal and because human beings are imperfect, but also because "moral passions," as Lionel Trilling notes, "are even more willful and imperious and impatient than the self-seeking passions." Dangers lurk in "our most generous wishes." Trilling continues, "Some paradox of our nature leads us, when once we have made our fellow men the objects of our enlightened interest, to go on to make them the objects of our pity, then of our wisdom, ultimately of our coercion." Thus, it is important to insist that a true community, involving equals, cannot exist without respect for persons, and that such respect requires procedures to protect rights as well as needs. Dax's case poses for us the challenge of trying to affirm both care and respect, community and individual rights, and to indicate how they

can be combined and which has priority when their conflict cannot
be avoided.

NOTES

1. For a fuller discussion of paternalism, see James F. Childress, *Who
Should Decide? Paternalism in Health Care* (New York: Oxford University
Press, 1982).

2. "A Happy Life Afterward Doesn't Make Up for Torture," *Washington
Post*, June 26, 1983.

3. Sharon Imbus and Bruce Zawacki, "Autonomy for Burn Patients
When Survival Is Unprecedented," *New England Journal of Medicine* 300
(August 1977): 308–11.

4. *Ten Years After a Severely Burned Patient's Request to Die: A Discussion
with Dax Cowart*. A videotape of "Medical Center Hour" at the University of
Virginia, Charlottesville, June 26, 1983.

5. "A Happy Life Afterward."

6. *Ten Years After.*

7. "A Happy Life Afterward."

8. *Ten Years After.*

Failed or Ongoing Dialogues?
Dax's Case 🕮 *Richard M. Zaner*

FEW IDEAS HAVE GRIPPED OUR MORAL IMAGINA-
tion more firmly than that of "rights." If we look into prevailing
moral discourse, either at the level of everyday moral life or that of
ethical theory, one finds an overwhelming number of issues whose
characteristic moral theme is said to be rights: of fetuses, infants,
children, adults, the elderly; of women, Blacks, those with Spanish
surnames, and other minorities; of the handicapped, the mentally
retarded, incompetents; of those needing organ transplants, those
with organs to donate; and on and on. If we take it seriously, there
are rights to health, birth, life, and death; to equal opportunity and
equal access; to receive medical care and to refuse it; to fair trial and
protection from crime; and countless others. The list is considerable, and the passion of their various advocates runs high.

When the person at issue is, like Dax Cowart, a patient severely compromised by illness or injury undergoing excruciating
pain (from the illness/injury, as from treatments), and who faces a
future so bleak it seems as if plotted by some deranged and agonized
soul, we then are forced to the realization of just how compelling
the appeal to rights can be. How could it possibly happen, Dax constantly implored, that in a society such as ours, whose moral focus is
so firmly set in the right of the individual to determine his or her

own course in life, precisely that right could at the same time be denied? An adult who was declared clearly competent and thus a person who just as clearly ought not be denied the right of self-determination, yet just this was in fact denied, and Dax was forced in the most literal way to undergo extraordinary and agonizing treatments against his own specific and declared wishes. Massively compromised in bodily abilities, profoundly and permanently disfigured, he was made to face a future devoid of everything he valued.

Such discourse is fueled by such commonly heard moral notions as "dignity," "respect," "beneficence," "personhood," "freedom of choice," and the like. As a people, we prize the "self-made" person: independent, self-reliant, self-determining, self-sufficient, the one who "did it my way" and "did it on my own." It is thus widely believed that respect for the individual is absolutely essential for understanding, evaluating, and deciding practically every medical-ethical issue. Theoretically advocated from many points of view, this notion serves as one of the basic rationales for a number of what are commonly thought to be key requirements of decision making: informed consent, for instance, or truth telling. It is central in complicated discussions concerning the right course to take in abortion, euthanasia, the use of placebos or double-blind techniques in human experimentation, and proxy decision making for incompetents.

The idea of "respect" extends further. A person is said to have the right to his or her own body and therefore to have control over what is done or not done to it. If we were to ask why we should respect another person or what it is that legitimates the idea that each of us has the right to choose, the widely accepted response is that underlying all of these ideas and rights is the core concept of moral order itself: each individual is a "free" and "autonomous" being, and this alone must be presupposed if any discussion about human conduct is to make sense.[1]

Immanuel Kant forcefully asserted this central thesis of modern individualism:

> The *autonomy* of the will is the sole principle of all moral
> laws and of the duties conforming to them; *heteronomy* of
> choice, on the other hand, not only does not establish my
> obligation but is opposed to the principle of duty and to
> the morality of the will. . . . [The] moral law expresses
> nothing else than the autonomy of the pure practical rea-
> son, i.e. freedom. This autonomy of freedom is itself the
> formal condition of all maxims, under which alone they
> can all agree with the supreme practical law.[2]

Morality makes no sense unless the person is autonomous. This is
the sole requirement without which human conduct can be neither
moral nor immoral.

It is little wonder that Dax's repeated appeal to his right to decide for himself is so compelling for our moral sensibility. We feel
strongly that it simply is not right for a person to be subjected to
anything neither chosen nor wished for. This, we sense, is a totally
unjustified intrusion into the freedom that constitutes us as moral
beings in the first place. To breech that barrier is to breech our very
humanity. No matter how much you or I might do or choose differ-
ently from Dax, it is plainly wrong to impose our own beliefs or
wishes onto him and force him to live a life he does not freely choose
to live, however much you or I might be ready to do so.

Even if, in a word, our "heroic" measures—the multiple skin
graft surgeries, the use of the Hubbard tank, the operations on his
eyes and hands, and the rest of what Dax had to go through—could
save a life, we must first of all consider whether by so doing we have
thereby made it necessary that only a hero could live that life. While
we cherish heroes, it is surely no part of our duties to force another
person to be one. And the rationale for all this, it is commonly believed, is that the adult, competent, rational person is an autonomous being governed solely by his or her own free will, "the sole
principle of all moral laws and of the duties conforming to them."
Dax and Dax alone, acting solely from his own free will, has the
right to decide whether to be treated.

Dax's case is compelling. The issue he raises is not trifling, for what is at stake is apparently the definitive feature of the moral order. We can thus appreciate Engelhardt's careful comment about the Cowart case, based on the videotape *Please Let Me Die*:

> When the patient who is able to give free consent does not, the moral issue is over. . . . In short, one must be willing, as a price for recognizing the freedom of others, to live with the consequences of that freedom: some persons will make choices that they would regret were they to live longer. But humans are not only free beings, but temporal beings, and the freedom that is actual is that of the present. Competent adults should be allowed to make tragic decisions, if nowhere else, at least concerning what quality of life justifies the pain and suffering of continued living. It is not medicine's responsibility to prevent tragedies by denying freedom, for that would be the greater tragedy. [3]

In the more recent film, *Dax's Case*, Cowart reaffirms his earlier decision, thereby giving ample credence to Engelhardt's point: we are free, but also temporal, and "the freedom that is actual is that of the present," whatever the future entailed by our present choices.

On the other side of things, of course, are the physicians, Dax's family (especially his mother), his attorney, Rex Houston, and doubtless others, who, however sympathetic and sensitive to his condition and future, refused to comply. If Dax's story is interpreted as that of autonomy and its compromise, then this other side is probably that of paternalism. Considered from the perspective of autonomy, and in perhaps the best light, this seems little more than a case of that well-known path paved with good intentions. These physicians, to speak only of them here, meant well and cared for Dax, but their actions were grievously mistaken and spelled but continued misery for him. Taken in its worst light, such paternalism seems a veritable bête noire: while physicians tried to prevent tragedy by continued treatment, their actions in effect denied

Dax his freedom, hence his personhood and autonomy, and thus caused an even greater tragedy by violating the moral order itself.

Of course, from the physicians' point of view, such paternalism (if that is what it was) is neither misleading, mistaken, nor an instance of cruelty. Indeed, they clearly insisted throughout that their personal moral outlook in effect be given its proper name— not paternalism, or if that then correctly understood, i.e., unselfish altruism, charity, humaneness, sympathy, goodness of heart, in short benevolence in a full sense. That it is often and unkindly interpreted as merely "good intentions" is unfortunate, but that does not imply that these physicians were either cruel or insensitive, unsympathetic or immoral. Indeed, they seem to say in the film (as Dr. White clearly displays in the earlier videotape *Please Let Me Die*), not only the historically embedded Hippocratic moral tradition— "love of one's fellowmen"[4]—but also present-day society obliges them to act on behalf of their patients' best interests, which they are often forced to interpret according to their own best lights.

Sociolegal and historical authorization and the sheer remarkable power of medicine to intervene effectively against disease and injury, it might be pointed out, is couched within a typical, taken for granted understanding of the relationship with patients, which almost invariably includes certain questionable assumptions about the effects of illness or injury and pain on the patient's ability to know and even to feel clearly what his or her own best interests actually are. Thus, physicians often assume that a person as severely injured as Dax, and who constantly experiences such extreme pain (whether from injuries, the treatments, or both), simply cannot know clearly what is best for him. It is indeed often noted that seriously burned patients regularly voice the very demands Dax did— that it is preferable to die than suffer treatment any longer, especially given the meager quality of life awaiting them even after the horrible pains are relieved. On the other hand, competency for many physicians is just not appropriately assessable until and if a patient is relieved from the pain and attains a more balanced view of the future. But the case could be made even more compelling, for even if Dax were competent, his demand not to be treated ran contrary to the basic moral norms governing medical practice, both historically and sociolegally. Compliance with his demand could only result in massive infections and a horrible death, while treatment could result in real potential for a productive life. The decision to treat thus seemed utterly obvious, reasonable, and necessary.

Thus understood, if Dax's physicians were paternalistic, it was not, from their point of view, a simple usurpation or violation of freedom or autonomy. It was an effort to help restore significant autonomy to him. In other words, it is only with an eye on the future that one can really and appropriately assess whether a patient's exercise of his or her actual (present) freedom should be accepted. It is thus not at all so obvious that it is freedom exercised in the present which is the significant sense, as Engelhardt, and apparently Dax, believe. Nor is it obvious that when "a patient who is able to give consent does not, the moral issue is over" (Engelhardt). Every exercise of free choice, it may be observed, is a decision for some future and against a range of others. It therefore always involves some set of reasons which, presumably, sway toward or support the future chosen and against those rejected. Whatever else "reasons" may signify, they are surely at least open for discussion, and not only (or only rarely) by the one deciding. Hence, when Dax refused to give his consent, the moral issue was far from being over. It has just begun; or, perhaps more accurately, the moral discourse has then been transformed dialogically. Now, a different sort of moral discussion has been initiated.

The reason for this is not hard to find. Any refusal of treatment, like a choice to be treated, inherently involves other people, physicians primarily. Every such choice by a patient invites a quite specific relationship with physicians. It also requires a set of specific actions (to do or not do, as the case may be) by these others. Having opted for a certain future (a demand to die by not being treated), Dax's choice necessarily requires that his physicians not only endorse and agree with the future tied to that choice, but even more that they actively and willingly participate in bringing it about. Indeed, in Dax's case, only someone else could bring it about.

The point is obvious: that a patient freely chooses not to consent to treatment does not close moral discussion (much less medical discussion), even though it surely does close out one phase of it. For now, as that choice ineluctably demands a specific decision and subsequent action by the physicians—i.e., compliance, hence not treating—the patient's choice essentially opens up a new phase of moral (and medical) discourse. It is an inherent feature of Dax's demand that he himself then engage in that further dialogue, that he be open (as he certainly seemed to have been) to the physician's questions and probings of among other things his reasons for refusing to consent. This must be done if for no other reason than that the physician is being asked as well to choose and act. Such choices and actions cannot be expected without further discussion, for the physician can no more be coerced than can Dax, as both are moral agents and so long as moral order is to be preserved. Thus, a patient who, after freely refusing consent, then should refuse as well to listen to physicians and to continue the dialogue, is as guilty of violating the moral order as a physician would be were he or she to refuse to listen to the patient, reflect on that, and in turn speak his or her own mind.

Several aspects of Dax's situation in 1974, then, are truly tragic. In the first place, whereas many patients, even some who are grievously ill or injured, can still "vote with their feet"—simply discharge their physicians and leave the scene on their own—Dax literally could not do that. For his choice to be realized, he had to rely on the actual participation of someone else—if not his physician, then another—who, had he or she so acted, would thereby be exposed to serious legal and moral consequences. For Dax's demand to be realized, on the other hand, there seems no alternative but that he also bear at least partial responsibility, however that be assessed, of that exposure. Neither in the videotape nor in the film, however, did Dax ever seem to want another person to become so exposed (although prior to transfer to Galveston, a physician agreed to his wish, with medical treatment reinstituted only after Dax's rapid, painful decline).

At the same time, though, it may well be that inability to leave the hospital on his own which gave the tragedy a further dimension. As long as he remained in the hospital, the pressures to continue treatment (at least until he could leave on his own) had to be intense. While hospitals may often seem to be "palaces of compulsive healing," in J. H. van den Berg's pithy phrase,[5] it also has to be recognized that they exist under considerable legal, social, and political pressure to be precisely that. We do not have institutions designed to manage patients such as Dax, for not even a hospice could legitimately accept him. Only those who are terminal, dying in spite of treatment, are hospice candidates. So long as Dax remained there, then, continued treatment was surely much easier, possibly even inevitable.

The other feature of his situation that seems profoundly tragic has to do with the way its moral tenor was construed, especially by Dax himself (but also, following that and its forceful presentation on the video, not to mention its repetition on the recent film, by many who saw and discussed the issue). Dax's choice not to consent is essentially one among many phases of an ongoing moral dialogue and has the effect of transforming it to a new phase. It inherently elicits the notice of others and moreover invites—even requires—response; specifically, it creates a situation of necessary, equally free choice and subsequent action on the part of the physician (among many other persons who must also, and in fact did, at some point enter the dialogue—family, friends, attorneys, nurses, other physicians, administrators, hospital boards, etc.).

Moral discourse is essentially dialogical, communal if you will. However, by framing the moral issues in the language of rights, Dax's demand inevitably elicited the response of an opposing right. Physicians, too, as well as those others, also have rights, equal and compelling in their way, precisely because they, too, must freely choose and act, hence assume responsibility. One right evokes (even provokes) opposing rights. To frame the issues in this way is to invoke the notion of autonomy, and this, similarly, tended to shape the physician's (and others') response as paternalism.

In such a situation, inevitable and unresolvable rivalry and conflict ensue, there being, as MacIntyre has shown,[6] no culturally or logically compelling way by which to weigh and resolve the multiple claims inherent to the rivaling viewpoints. Such a situation is a plain and deeply tragic *a-poria*—a "no exit." It thus becomes almost fateful that the continuation of treatment gets construed as paternalistic in the worst sense, i.e., as the more or less sheer exercise of power by the physician and the hospital. To construe the moral situation in this way is to make it at best adversarial, a situation in which someone has to be right and someone else wrong. And that destroys the dialogical character of moral discourse. The moral order, far from being revealed by or based on such notions as autonomy and rights, is thereby violated.

This points to the centering issue Dax's case poses. As with every profound and tragic moral dilemma, did it really have to be that way back in 1974? Were there no ways at hand for promoting and sustaining the moral dialogue? Indeed, did the dialogues actually fail? While the tragedy itself remains hauntingly with us, marking out a moral failure by many of us to understand the exigencies of moral dialogue (as well as the many traps and snares in its path), much can be learned about it, and other cases, by viewing them in the framework of dialogue. And this means dialogue itself must be a principal topic of moral reflection.

Consider the following a kind of palimpsest on dialogue as a moral adventure.[7] First, something of a digression to set the stage.

In William Golding's novel, *Lord of the Flies*,[8] the marooned children quickly form a kind of society governed by rules, led by the clever Ralph, a society kept constantly in check by the awful presence of, and the ritualized ceremonies focused about, "the Beast" on the island's hill. One of the boys, Simon, after a searing encounter with the children-tribe's gift to pacify the beast—a pig's head impaled on a stake—makes his way painfully through creepers and thickets, over difficult boulders, up the cliff to the top of the hill. It was not that he had that in mind nor planned to go up there to confront the Beast. It was not that at all; only, "What else is there to do?" Weary, staggering, he reaches the top and, buffeted by the winds, sees a "flicker of blue stuff against brown clouds." Pushing on, he sees a "humped thing suddenly sit up" and look down at him. Hiding his face, he toils on: "The flies had found the figure too. The life-like movement would scare them off for a moment so that they made a dark cloud round the head. Then as the blue material of the parachute collapsed the corpulent figure would bow forward, sighing, and the flies settle once more." [9]

He understands: a parachutist (it is wartime) had fallen (probably already near death, his plane shot down) and his parachute had become hung in the high rocks atop the hill. As the wind caught the parachute, it flailed out the man's limbs. The "Beast" is but that! Simon's first reactions are to examine the bones, flesh, "the colours of corruption," pitilessly held together by the layers of rubber of his flying suit and the canvass of the harness. The putrid odor gets to be too much and he vomits. Then, feeling pity for the "poor body that should be rotting away," he frees the parachute lines from the rocks "and the figure from the wind's indignity." We should note this first reaction, the turn, in pity and sympathy, toward the pilot even though dead and putrid smelling.

Having restored what dignity he could to the body, he surveys the scene on the beach below, and sees the other boys had shifted their camp away from the hill, away from the "Beast," and had made their sacrificial offering. Then a curious thing happens: "As Simon thought this [the shift of the camp], he turned to the poor broken thing that sat stinking by his side. The beast was harmless and horrible; and the news must reach the others as soon as possible." [10]

Why this thought, right after his redignifying the corpse and before anything else occurred to him? Simon apparently does nothing from a sense of personal pride; he seeks neither reward, nor fame, nor power. Indeed, he alone (although possibly also his intellectual friend, Piggy) seems to have a clear grasp of the realities of the little society, a Leviathan in miniature. Hence, he might well be said to know already pretty much what he will get into, once he's back down the hill with his news. He simply says, "The news must reach the others." And, when he finally staggers down towards the camp, it is already night, and the boys, already whipped into a craze by Ralph, are dancing and chanting, "Kill the beast! Cut his throat! Spill his blood!" A storm has come up on the horizon, shattering the sky with periodic, hammering light and blasting noise, and the boys (a "throb and stamp of a single creature") suddenly see a thing crawling out of the forest at the foot of the hill: "Him! Him!" and they set upon it with sticks, beating, crunching its bones, biting and tearing its flesh. On its knees, arms folded over its face, it "was crying out against the abominable noise something about a body on a hill."

It is, of course, Simon who is brutalized and killed. For all this, nevertheless, there is Simon's lucid moment at the top of the hill: his move toward the dead pilot to undo the indignity, his curious urge to "tell the others." Why? What is this turn toward the others, especially those who, it is clear in the story, are hardly sympathetic with Simon and his strange ways?

What needs to be held in mind here is telling the others, this need for "talk" or "speech" about what "things truly are." Golding's powerful tale reminds me of Plato's myth of the cave, and with that of the urge to dialogue, to speak ("say" and "listen") together, sharing what is one's own with the other. And, with that, too, of the Platonic *a-poria* so intrinsic to dialogue: the participant in dialogue at some point feels overcome or set upon, unable to continue to do (whatever it may be) or be (whatever he or she has been up to then), without stopping and thoughtfully dwelling within the happening of what, through dialogical speaking, has overcome him or her and obliged questioning. That is, he or she undergoes the concrete experience of not-knowing and wanting-to-know something deeply vital (ultimately, *himself* or *herself*), hence of questioning: asking, being challenged, doubting, exploring, unearthing—whatever it takes to resolve what has overcome him or her, or get free *from* not knowing and thus become free *for* genuine knowing and the right speech and action that must then follow.

To question, that is, to beseech, appeal, request; to seek response, and in the double sense, to seek what is *responsive* to one's realized ignorance or need to know (what speaks to it relevantly and truly), and to seek what is *responsible* (what can be counted on as truly resolving the question that led to the *a-poria*). To question is thus to open oneself up (or to find oneself already opened up by the question), to find oneself at the disposal of whatever responsively/ responsibly speaks to one's condition or quandary so as to permit movement out of the no exit. To question is to appeal to others (most often to other persons, but also to oneself taken as the other). It is an urgent seeking; the *a-poria* means that one can no longer do or be what one has done and been before; it is an appeal to others to share in one's own questioning. Thus, it is a telling (a significance and a sharing) of oneself to or before the others who are sought out as responders, indeed, as coseekers.

What about this invited response? Suppose one grants that the questioning is utterly genuine: Dax's deep puzzlement over his right to choose for himself is completely genuine and deeply felt. What about the response others make? Can anything guarantee that the other person will respond in the way the questioner seeks and needs responsively and responsibly? Can Dax demand that his physician respond, much less that, if there is a response, it will be as honest as the question? Merely because Dax's questions are authentic, does this of itself assure that there will be any response at all? What could possibly assure a person such as Dax (or any other severely injured/ill person) that others will surrender themselves to his issue, to what is at stake? Is it even possible nowadays for patients such as Dax and physicians to engage in a shared search for honest and courageous resolution as that exhibited back in 1974?

Or, even if there is an honest asking (telling-to-others, sharing, or wanting to share one's own *a-poria*), who will listen? What kind of sharing do Dax's pleas really invite? In a society in which there is such an aggressive heterogeneity of moral and religious points of view, and in which there are no ways (short of violence) of weighing their respective, rival claims on our actions and lives, various modes of violence seem if not the open agenda then surely not far from it.

And the problem lies at the root of dialogue, not so much with the initiator (the questioner) but the listener, precisely what Plato knew so well. Questioning, if you will, knows itself to be genuine, for the questioner really does not know and it is vital for him or her to know. The issue of dialogue is that the questioner cannot be assured in advance and in the same ways about the genuineness of the response, or even whether he or she will be listened to.

In the end, nothing assures that the patient will be actually listened to. Listening can only be itself a free act, invited by the questioner, never forced or in that sense demanded. To try to force response, much less a very specific response, is to vitiate the inner sense of the question since this only masquerades as genuine not-knowing and needing-to-know, hence it cuts the ground out from dialogue.

Nothing can bring about response, then, unless the other recognizes that the question is addressed to him or her and decides to respond. However, suppose that the other does respond for whatever reasons. Then, the inner demands of dialogue come into play: responding, the other person (physician) addresses the first (Dax), claims to address his appeal or quandary, and claims at least that the response is both responsive (to the issue at stake) and responsible (for the response given). Thus, the response is itself necessarily open to further questions, by Dax in the first place, but also possibly by others whose entrance into the dialogue signals their openness as well. It is, after all, the one who questions and who thus seeks to know, who needs to know and whose understanding and fate are at issue. Questions seek responses; when given, responses claim to be relevant, responsive, responsible, etc., to the question. But, whether the response is relevant, etc., requires further dialogue. That is, responses are taken up within the dialogue as mere claims, and as such are always to be tested. As claims, they are dialogically held in suspension or parentheses, held in abeyance precisely to enable this further dialogue, testing, by the one whose ignorance and inquiry is at issue. Thus, responses are essentially invitations to further questions, which lead to still further responses, to further questions, and so on—in shared talk (com-munication), until and if that point is reached when the dialogical partners are free from ignorance and freed for truth, that truth which resolves the *a-poria* and is thus freeing.

Obviously, at any moment the entire process of dialogue can break down, be betrayed, diverted, become aborted in many ways and for many reasons: failed insight, sloppy thinking and talk, dishonesty, impatience, and still others. But once initiated, dialogue—founded on honesty, restraint, and courage—is inherently exposed to such failures, and the failures reflect on those who make them by their own free choices, for that alone initiates the dialogue and sustains its course in shared discourse.

Such reflections, however, require that we not be naive. After all, just as Socrates, so all of us can and do use all manner of tricks, guises and disguises, cunning and cleverness, to make the invitation to listeners and readers as attractive and inviting as possible. The appeal needs to be appealing. But is not that only a guise covering over the exercise of power or manipulation? Can there be an appeal (a way of speaking, or writing) which is not also manipulation in one or another sense of violence, merely using the other person, hence coercing him or her in some way? More directly, is dialogue possible without manipulation (hence use of power, hence violence)? Or, what is the relationship between dialogue, as the form of moral discourse, and violence? Is Dax, in his very demand and emphasis on his own rights, being manipulative? Are his physicians, in their refusal to comply, being in turn manipulative even while attempting to carry on the dialogue with him? Is there anything which can assure us to the contrary of either?

At the heart of this is something very much like what Golding captures in the child, Simon: that quick turn to the pilot's indignity, that odd, forboding turn to the other children that the "news must be told." There is here what Alfred Schutz describes as a *Du-einstellung*, a being oriented to the other person.[11] But, whether that *Du-einstellung* will be unilateral (the other ignores me), reciprocal (the other orients himself or herself towards me, recognizes that I am asking), or mutual (the other dialogically responds), can only be a free act, since otherwise the initiating act of questioning is viti-ated—which may be the greater tragedy in Dax's case (no matter whose fault it may have been). Dax's free choice to refuse consent, in other words, is not merely telling other people what he wishes; it is more accurately an invitation for these others to respond freely and mutually, without force or violence, whatever the other may make of that invitation. It is, then, an act that seeks to enable the other to be free in his or her response (as authentic listening is an act enabling the question to be genuinely spoken), thereby enabling the questioner to be free from and free for. Thereby, too, the responder becomes freed. The dialogical partners who are able to sustain moral dialogue, thus, effectively collaborate in each other's free-dom, as Gabriel Marcel long ago emphasized.[12] Freedom is not the act of a solitary consciousness or pure will; it is rather the mutually enabling act which occurs, when and if it does occur, at the heart of moral dialogue.

Morality is therefore not a matter merely of autonomy; it is, rather, that of mutual enablement, an act of com-muning with one another about issues that matter, make a difference in one's life. Its hope is that the act of genuine questioning (Dax: Isn't it my right to decide for myself?) will really speak to or tell the other person, will in that sense be significant for the other who, hopefully, will really listen and then respond with the asker. But its hope is just as impor-tantly that the asker will take the response (Physician: But after all, what you are asking violates my own deeply held moral beliefs!) in the same way the asker asks the responder to do—that here, too, there will be real listening and talking with the responder. By shar-ing freely with the other, the hope is that that very act itself will enable the other (both Dax and the physician) to be responsive and responsible from within his or her own life, and will then be open for further seeking.

And what are we to make of the tricks, the devices, disguises, guises, and ironies of discourse? The centering issues here are at the nub of actual talk among people, ingredient to our naturally occurring conversations, our dialogue. Each of the participants in moral dialogue must continually and in every conduct and speech remind one another that they can each only be free to respond and to question. The "others must be told," but the telling must also be the awesome telling of the other that he or she is able to be, and must be, free, and in this freedom must be responsive and responsible.

The core response to the cunning and wiliness of reason is the moral one: the moral of a person's lifestory is within the moral dialogues of his or her life. If the questioner in any way masks or betrays the other's freedom to respond (prohibits, conceals, or disguises the other from this), and if the same is not true as well for the responder, then manipulation, power play, control, and violence are invariably at hand, and the morality of the discourse is destroyed. In different terms, it is only by both participants' continual and insistent enabling of each other to be themselves in speaking, only by displaying this in each of the respective "talkings," that freedom is at all possible. Each collaborates in the other's freedom and responsibility. Freedom is therefore not a matter of autonomy, but rather of mutuality.

It remains only to insist on this, that the one who questions, who initiates the moral dialogue, faces an ultimate test, perhaps anguish, the actual prospect of having to live in the face and in the aftermath of the other's choices. The same is true for the responder, that genuine listening and responding will itself go unheeded, whether the asker was merely playing around, looking for an answer of which he or she was already convinced, or whatever.

The same is true, too, of an author: to live with the real possibility that none will read his or her words; and for the teacher, that none will listen—that, in short, dialogue will not occur. How one can come to accept that and resist the very real temptation to use force on the listener/reader, however indirectly or subtly, is perhaps the awesome challenge to one's courage in sustaining dialogue with others about vital issues.

Although, in a way, the dialogues between Dax and his physicians (but also with his family, attorney, etc.) may have failed—or may have been thought to have failed—it must be recognized that in a number of important ways they did not fail, but were sustained over time, albeit in frequent pain and anguish on all their parts. Dax, though he did not get what he demanded, managed to resolve some of the issues; he has, indeed, even thrived in important ways in the aftermath of the events of 1973–74, despite what he seems inclined to think were failed dialogues back then. Dax did initiate a discourse back in 1974, and it was a moral dialogue. His physician, his mother, and his attorney, Rex Houston, on the other hand, did not vacate nor did they vitiate that dialogue; they rather engaged in it in the most direct ways, squarely confronting the issue Dax posed.

Especially in view of the film it must be said that when those dialogues seemed to have devolved into adversarial confrontation, pitting autonomy against presumed paternalism, the flaw may well have been Dax's. To judge from the film and my own conversations with him, despite the quite evident spiritual growth he exhibits in so many ways, his needle seems plainly stuck: "I was right, and should have been allowed to choose for myself." As suggested earlier, to construe the issue as one of rights seems willy-nilly to have foreclosed the essential openness dialogue needs in order to thrive and enrich its participants. On the other hand, it also seems necessary to recognize that what went wrong in 1974 was not at all that Dax's freedom was violated, but rather that the dialogue seems to have failed, or if not that, then surely to have been sorely compromised. Instead of mutually enabling discourse, aggressive adversaries were created by pitting autonomy against paternalism.

Finding the dialogue at a kind of impasse, it is revealing to reflect on what Dax then did—make his case on video. Dax spoke to other health professionals, especially those still in training—not simply to urge them to simplistic acceptance of a patient's every whim and desire, but rather to learn to respect a person, accomplished most concretely and existentially through common discourse, the vehicle of moral dialogue. Dax's efforts here, it cannot be ignored, were, and continue to be, extraordinarily sensitive to the dilemmas such patients as he present to physicians. But neither can it be forgotten that this significant dialogical step was initiated and videotaped by one of his physicians, Dr. White, who, like others of his physicians, was and continues to be uncommonly sensitive to the plight of patients such as Dax.

Please Let Me Die can be interpreted as one way by which this moral dialogue could continue, even when direct talk seemed at an impasse. It underscores the enormous significance of ongoing talk between patients and physicians as the primary means by which patient trust and confidence may be achieved. Its initiation by Dr. White also underscores and powerfully symbolizes the need by patients to be responsibly responsive to the morality at the heart of medical practice. The physician's care of and for patients needs to be concretely textured by actual concern of the sort which everyday talk seems uniquely capable of achieving in such cases as this.

In the same way, *Dax's Case* is a continuation of this dialogue, although its issues are far broader. For now, the key theme is centered on the existential aftermath of the case and is a dialogical invitation for viewers to engage in the most concrete ways with Dax in understanding what happens to patients after discharge. In a word, his continued initiating of dialogues in another form—a possibility opened up and enabled by others, including physicians—is quite remarkable. This film and that early video stand as a significant invitation for others to engage in a dialogue with him over issues that bring a human life into ever so sharp a focus.

NOTES

1. H. Tristram Engelhardt, Jr., "Basic Ethical Principles in the Conduct of Biomedical and Behavioral Research Involving Human Subjects,"

The Belmont Report, The National Commission for the Protection of Human Subjects of Biomedical and Behavioral Research, DHEW Publication No. (OS) 78-0013 (Washington, D.C.: U.S. Government Printing Office, 1978), 3.

2. Immanuel Kant, *Critique of Practical Reason*, tr. I. W. Beck (Indianapolis: Bobbs-Merrill Press, 1956), 33–34.

3. H. Tristram Engelhardt, Jr., "A Demand to Die," *Hastings Center Report* 5 (June 1975): 47.

4. See L. Edelstein, *Ancient Medicine* (Baltimore: Johns Hopkins University Press, 1967), 337–47.

5. J. H. van den Berg, *Medical Power and Medical Ethics* (Pittsburgh: Duquesne University Press, 1978), 4.

6. Alasdair MacIntyre, *After Virtue* (Notre Dame: Notre Dame Press, 1981).

7. *Palimpsest:* (1) "paper, parchment, etc., prepared for writing on and wiping out again . . . "; (2) "A parchment, etc., which has been written upon twice, the original writing having been rubbed out" (*Oxford English Dictionary*). Latin *palimpsestus* from Greek *palimpsēstos*, "rubbed again": *palin*, "again . . . ", *psēstos*, "scraped"; from *psēn*, "to rub," "scrape."

8. William Golding, *Lord of the Flies* (New York: Capricorn Books, 1955).

9. Ibid., 181.

10. Ibid.

11. See Alfred Schutz, *The Structures of the Life-World*, I, tr. H. Tristram Engelhardt, Jr., and Richard M. Zaner (Evanston, Ill.: Northwestern University Press, 1973), 61–64.

12. Gabriel Marcel, *Le mystère de l'être*, I, Aubier (Paris: Editions Montaigne, 1951), 144.

Dax's Case: Management Issues in Medicine ⚕ *Joanne Lynn*

DAX COWART IS A WONDERFUL, FORCEFUL, CApable person. And he did not wish to be alive to tell his story. He is alive only because very well-meaning family, friends, and health care personnel did not heed his request to be allowed to die. His life now is rewarding, even pleasant. Yet Dax says he should not be alive.

The film documenting his story is extraordinarily powerful. Interspersed with his narration of the events and his evaluations are interviews with the other key figures who provided his care. They are personable, likeable, honest people giving quite candid and unguarded views. To its credit, the film never makes them look silly or cruel. In fact, the film never makes a clear statement of who, if anyone, was wrong.

For me, the film raises two substantial, interrelated issues. First, beyond legal rights and adversary language, how should Dax have been treated by the responsible care givers? Second, if good management led to a demand to be killed, should physicians be authorized to do so? Only with a full understanding of the question of euthanasia can the question of competent management be addressed. But also, competent management requires clear understanding of the merits and the availability of death-seeking care plans.

63

CASE MANAGEMENT

Dax's case was badly mismanaged, and the two major physicians involved did not even seem to learn anything from their errors. The physician in charge is, after all, just that—in charge. Especially in a situation like this where the patient is so severely disabled and dependent, the attending physician has the role-related responsibility to attend to all of the patient's concerns, not just his physiological derangements. Ordinarily, in order to do that, physicians must grant to patients the authority to govern their lives as they see fit. Some patients will gladly return this authority to the physician or displace it to a family member. But it must be clear from the outset and throughout health care that the patient can maintain or recover the authority to make whatever choices can be made.

Surely Dax Cowart should have had a way to extricate himself from the lifesaving treatment he was getting. Surely it is an outrage that one physician bypassed getting his consent because he could not physically sign a form, and another freely admits ignoring Dax's protests. One might even wish that Dax had sued these jailguard/doctors for false imprisonment and for the costs of care.

But whether this case was mismanaged is the easy question. The harder questions arise in trying to rewrite the story. How should Dax's case have been managed?

Emergency Care

One cannot fault the kindly farmer who refused to get a rifle when he first found the severely burned young man along the road. Likewise, the ambulance attendants who brought him to the first and then the second hospital must have the authority to try to save even those who protest, for the emergency does not permit evaluation of competence, time for information exchange, or even personalized assessment of likely future possibilities. There are some protests against treatment in emergency settings which should be honored, but we can hardly expect ambulance workers in the field regularly to be the arbiters of this issue. Even the physicians at Parkland Hospital in the first few hours are largely exempt from obtaining adequate consent for their treatment.

However, very shortly the situation changes. Depending somewhat on physiologic and psychologic stability of the patient, sometime in the first few days his views about the desirability of various outcomes become important. Thus, from very early in the case, Dax must start getting accurate information about the possible futures—not just the most hopeful, but also the median results and the real options, including nontreatment.

Biases and Ambiguities

Sometimes, perhaps often, physicians deliberately obfuscate or mislead in providing information. Certainly, they often withhold information of crucial importance. In general, manipulating the patient by misleading through the information received is indefensible dishonesty. The only valid defenses are: (1) an accommodation of the patient's clear preference to avoid some information and some direct responsibility for choices or (2) an avoidance of cruelty and suffering by arranging the timing and setting of information giving so as to be most manageable by the patient. Neither of these applies to a patient such as Dax. The patient wanted information and time and opportunity were available.

However, a somewhat different error may actually be more common—the physician does not know accurate prognostic information. Even for burn injuries where the number of centers is small and the literature fairly manageable, it would probably be very difficult to give Dax even an accurate statistical projection of the likelihood and nature of various critical outcomes. What were the real chances of saving vision, of restoring any hand function, of walking, of self-care? What suffering would each require, and how much time would it take?

If the data here are anywhere near as fragmentary as in most of medicine, the answers are exceedingly imprecise. We can probably say whether any particular outcome is possible as a theoretical matter (or are the necessary anatomic and physiologic components absent?) and whether it has ever been achieved (or is it unprecedented?). But that is far different from being able to give an honest "median and standard deviation" for each important end point. Yes, Dax could survive, maybe was even likely to survive, but how many with burns like his did not and what happened to them? Maybe some hand function could conceivably be restored, but how likely was it to achieve various functions? If I were in his situation, I would want to have a lot of information of this type. As a physician, I know that I ordinarily do not have that sort of information to give.

There needs to be more research on what happens with various situations and choices. I once was called to testify as to whether a woman with admittedly diminished mental abilities, could refuse amputation of a gangrenous leg.[1] Obviously, one needs to know what would happen if there were no amputation. The medical literature offered nothing that applied to her situation. At trial, one set of physicians claimed that she would die within the next few weeks without the amputation. Another set reported that they knew of some contrary cases, living for a year or more. The patient kept the leg and died of another cause six months later. But, when her situation arises again, once again the medical prognostication will be filled with bias and anecdote—not because anyone thinks that is better than comprehensive descriptions of matched series receiving different treatments, but because the better data are not available.

Required Information

What information should have been provided to Dax? Certainly it should give as honest a portrayal of his future as his physicians could construct, along with the most optimistic of possibilities and some intelligible expressions of the degree of reliability of all the information.

Also, he should have been told of the process of care in the hospital. Who determines the plan of care and how? Would he have any choice among hospitals or physicians or nurses or therapists? How could he protest? What would be his mother's and his lawyer's roles? What could happen if he wanted nonstandard treatment? What rights and responsibilities would the law enforce? What options might legal considerations bar? What options might be legal but probably could not be exercised in a particular hospital setting?

Obviously, not all of this information should be given at one time or in one way. It should be given responsively to the patient's questions and concerns. But enough should be given to ensure that the patient understands his or her medical condition and the workings of this unfamiliar social system and to ensure that he or she is empowered to make those choices that can be made available, which always include not being treated.

Within the first week or two, with a reasonably competent patient who wishes to be involved in the choices, the patient should know most of what is known about likely outcomes, what will have to be gone through in order to achieve various outcomes, and how his or her requests will be honored or challenged. The patient should have some opportunity, if at all possible, to agree to a care team.

Management of Early Refusal of Treatment

What should be done if the patient objects to treatment in the early stages, after the extreme emergency of the first twenty-four to forty-eight hours and before the patient and the key care givers are well known to one another? The responsible physician should bargain for time. Nearly all patients are willing to enter a time-limited agreement. Nearly any suffering is more tolerable if there is a clear end point. Dax Cowart has told me that he thinks he would have been quite willing to make such a bargain with a physician. In the time agreed upon, the physician could seek to modify the care plan maximally so as to make it meet the patient's concerns. In Dax's case, that at least would have meant to treat his pain more vigorously and to have him meet with survivors who have done well.

This meeting with those who have gone before is one aspect of information giving that medicine has been exceedingly slow in employing. Maybe some people really think in statistical terms about their bodies and lives, but most of my patients and friends really seem to use (or to construct) "stories" of how things will work out. We may well use the statistics in constructing such stories, but it is the story itself that we "try on for fit" and see if certain kinds of futures are "better fits" than are others. Nothing is so powerful in projecting oneself into futures than meeting or even reading about or hearing about people who have traveled a road quite similar to one's own.

What should be done if the patient, who is an adult and is not adjudicated incompetent and is beyond the first few days, will not bargain and will not accept treatment which the physician regards as essential? Then and only then are the care givers, family, and patient forced to rely on legal rights and responsibilities. The responsible physician, presumably in consultation with the rest of the care team, must decide two issues: (1) whether the patient might be incompetent and (2) whether the care the patient prefers can and should be available in their care setting. If there is a question of competence, the physician must seek an expedited court response to the question while trying to give what care can be supplied.

Conscience-Based Disputes

Whether or not the patient is competent to make choices, the care givers and even the institution can ordinarily choose not to be party to certain choices made by the patient or a court-appointed surrogate. While most of the conscience clauses in institutional health care practice have grown up around abortion, the same logic applies to exempting, in general, individual providers and institutions from courses of conduct they feel to be immoral. (Of course, this does not readily extend to justifying an exemption because the conduct is potentially financially disadvantageous or has troublesome effects upon public image.) Thus, if a patient or a duly appointed surrogate wishes to pursue a course of action that is legal, but not acceptable to the patient's care-giving team or institution, the patient must be assisted in transferring to another setting.

If that is not possible, then some compromise or arbitration must be worked out. This is an honest dilemma, with all parties bearing equally strong claims. While the disadvantaged position of the patient often argues for some bias in favor of protecting the patient's claims over the provider's, in real situations the wise answer will have to come from careful consideration of the facts and circumstances of each individual case.

Bargains and Time-Limited Trials

If, however, a bargain has been struck between patient and physician to defer a decision against life-sustaining treatment for a period of time, then the care givers have a responsibility to live up to its terms, even if the outcome is adverse to the provider's preferences. Perhaps the patient is considered to be competent and agrees to a one-month trial of therapy with the proviso that, if it fails *in the patient's assessment,* he or she will have the authority to stop lifesaving treatment and die, and the care-giving team will continue to provide effective symptom relief and bodily care. A care-giving team would be unfair not to follow through on its promise. If a new question of competence arises during the trial period, that may warrant brief delay for resolution, but it does not warrant callous disregard of the prior agreement.

Often, time-limited trials are advantageous even when the patient (or surrogate) feels the treatment is definitely indicated. I now rarely start a respirator, feeding tube, or dialysis without simultaneously establishing a schedule for reassessment of the merits. Too many times care givers, patients, and families find it far easier to continue whatever treatments have been started than to change. Often a treatment has outlasted its merits, but no one can readily point out that fact. Time-limited trials create that opportunity.

Role of Family of Competent Patient

What should be the roles of the family of a competent patient? To have put Dax's mother in the position of rubber stamp for the doctor's wishes and antagonist with her son is inexcusable. The first physician even said that she was the correct person because Dax could not physically sign the form! One wonders what the doctor would have done if Dax had no family, or had they all spoken a foreign language. Clearly, Dax's mother was—and is—very important to him. But she should never have been allowed to enforce his confinement or to feel responsible for his choices. She hoped he would accept his religious responsibilities before he died, but surely someone could have talked with her about the necessity of him accepting Christ voluntarily. Surely, someone in the hospital could have counseled her as to the possibility that she need not feel responsible for Dax's salvation, and that she certainly was not responsible for decisions affecting his physical health. She had just lost her husband; compassion alone would dictate that physicians should not encourage her to feel responsible for keeping her son alive.

If she had thought it incorrect for the physician to accept Dax's directive to be allowed to die, she should be empowered to seek review of his competence or the legality of his behavior. But she should never have been given the authority to make choices contravening his own without due process for Dax.

Outcomes

So, what should have been the outcome for Dax? Should he, as he has claimed both then and now, have been allowed to die of overwhelming sepsis? I hope it would not have worked out that way. I hope Dax would have chosen to survive. No one can know whether he would have. Certainly, he would have borne the responsibility for his choices. Instead of railing at his captors, he would have to face the lonely, sometimes awesome, responsibility for really making the choices. Maybe the situation would still look unchanged: such severe suffering now and such severe permanent disability that the treatments to save life were not warranted. But perhaps the pause that is ordinarily engendered by the knowledge that his directive would be followed, would have led Dax to accept treatment, though perhaps grudgingly, piecemeal, and with anger at fate. Certainly, this is what many people experience.

And how should his care givers, family, and friends respond to his choice? People in that community of care might best seek honest, respectful, humble, and passionate responses. There need be no particular bias toward life or toward accepting death, though any individual certainly may have and ordinarily may express his or her views. But, finally, we must each be willing to serve others and to let them refuse our service.

EUTHANASIA

What should happen if Dax had chosen to die and if dying with any reasonable comfort required the assistance of others? Should physicians and nurses be allowed to act so as to assure death?

We must first acknowledge that choices now routinely shape how and when people die. One can well imagine that this was true in the past—George Washington no doubt died from the leechings as much as from his illness—but the situation was not seen in this way. Perhaps the infrequency of a clear causal relationship and more ready acceptance of the power of fate allowed people to deny that treatment choices were responsible for death, blaming only their bad fortune.

Legal Prohibitions

Of course, God or nature cannot be punished when responsible for cutting short a person's life, so homicide, suicide, and civil liability issues do not arise when the facts are constructed in this way. However, death usually now follows prolonged chronic illnesses, offering many opportunities for interventions, each of which is expected to cause both benefits and harms. People can no longer readily escape responsibility for their choices. The older interpretation would find anyone who is responsible for shortening a person's life guilty of murder, assisted suicide, or suicide, and also liable for any resultant civil damages. "The law of this state does not allow anyone to shorten another's life. . . . The morality of the defendant's conduct, the purity of their motives, common practice in this type of situation, and the wishes of the decedent's family are all of no weight."[2]

Modern ethical writings regarding decision making[3] would authorize patients and their surrogates to balance the likely length of life offered by each treatment choice against other attributes of the life obtained. That is, Dax should have been able to choose to avoid pain or disability even if thereby his life were shortened. The current understanding of good medical treatment and the traditional interpretation of the legal and moral responsibility for death then come into conflict, for what one wants to consider good practice might be punishable under homicide or assisted suicide charges.

The conflict is not easily resolved. Maintaining a strict construction of the legal responsibilities to avoid homicide and assisted suicide would force lives of great suffering to be extended and even worsened, despite the objections of the sufferers and the brutalization of care givers. This course was actually inflicted upon Dax. On the other hand, if society were free to condone early death from medical treatment decisions, then some people—perhaps many people—would die when they should have been treated. What one would want, obviously, is to require and allow only the right decisions, but to maintain severe penalties for those who effectuate erroneous decisions that result in an earlier death. This is exceedingly difficult.

What should count as correct or incorrect decisions is expected to vary greatly for different people. Two patients with exactly Dax's physical condition could have personal value commitments and concerns that would lead to maximally aggressive life-sustaining care being correct for one (and less painful or burdensome treatments being seriously in error) while the reverse is true for the other. Thus, dividing acceptable from unacceptable decisions cannot depend simply upon the physiological outcome but must also reflect the patient's particular characteristics and evaluation of the merits of various outcomes. This goal can only be achieved if it is internalized by the medical and nursing professions. The substance of such a complex assessment can only have a pallid reflection in statute or regulation. Furthermore, assessments of the merits of outcomes are much too frequent and too private to allow for external review and affirmation of each one without incurring unacceptable costs in resource utilization, delay, and loss of privacy.

Instead, the law enforces the honoring of some elements of a process aimed at ensuring patient participation and at protecting patient's rights, which shape the first section of this paper, and the law bars killing (or assisting in the suicide of) patients. Yet choosing medical treatment options that lead to a shorter life is commonplace, criminal prosecutions are so rare as to be aberrations,[4] and civil liability in this setting is also exceedingly infrequent. People confronted with these situations have developed practical solutions that do seem to be able to balance the relevant considerations appropriately. Health care professionals and the public seem to concur that some kinds of choices are not what was meant to be considered murder (or even a source of liability under tort or contract law). The choice of a dying cancer patient to decline one more transfusion or operation occasions sympathy and compassion but not outrage. However, if a physician were to shoot a patient, even if motivated by compassion, that would be met with outrage—and with murder charges.

These moral sentiments are rarely defended with careful analysis. In fact, the phrases used to express them are often quite imprecise and inconsistent when applied to difficult and ambiguous cases. Definitions cannot be clear, descriptive, and objective and still compare with ordinary usage for common terms such as "terminal illness," "extraordinary treatment," or "allowing to die," largely because such terms express a conclusion regarding the correctness of a treatment choice more than they give a reason for the conclusion. Nowhere is this more evident than in the description of the cause of a person's death.[5] Dax's death after stopping treatment would have had multiple causes, including the fact of human mortality, the choices to stop life-extending treatment, and the choices to encourage complications by going home. Saying that a person died from a particular disease conveys the conclusion that no one is to be held responsible for the death, even if the time and manner of death is the result of deliberate choices as well as the natural forces. Saying that the cause of death was certain actions of a person's physician conveys that the physician is to be held responsible, even if the natural course of disease was not altered. Thus, the use of the term "cause of death," which many people perceive as descriptive and morally neutral, is actually quite evaluative, though it conveys the conclusion rather than the evaluation itself.

Other ambiguities in these phrases abound, but it remains striking that they are so commonly used. Clearly, they are helping people to draw lines between acceptable and unacceptable behavior in ways that ordinarily suffice. In difficult cases, it may be appropriate to look behind the ordinary usage for the underlying moral justification. For example, in a case involving the desirability of artificial nutrition or antibiotics, it becomes important to see that "extraordinary" treatment is not really "statistically infrequent" nor "artificial and intrusive," but is actually any treatment that offers benefits so small that they are disproportionate to the burdens imposed.[6]

Policy Considerations

However, this analysis and clarification may not always be the important thing to do. Some distinctions are not directly rooted in morally relevant considerations but rather in the pragmatic consideration that adopting the admittedly problematic distinction leads to a better society than would rejecting it. This, I believe, is the case with the distinction between active steps that end life and passive steps that allow death to come. Although the distinction is clear enough in some cases, in many which description should be applied is ambiguous. Would stopping Dax's antibiotics count as an active interruption of an ongoing process or a passive desisting to allow death to come? Furthermore, the categorization as active or passive does not correlate perfectly with the acceptability of the steps taken. Some active steps that shorten life are obligatory—consider the giving of morphine to consenting persons suffering from the last stages of some painful cancers. And some passive steps that allow life to end early are morally reprehensible—consider the deliberate failure even to try to save Dax from the start, especially if rooted in financial considerations.

The Case Against Active Killing

Maintaining a very firm stand against active steps that overtly lead to an earlier death, even while permitting many passive "allowings to die," seems to be the social policy. The "passive" choices, so long as freely chosen or clearly in the patient's interest or both, are now readily accepted by most physicians, commentators, and patients. However, active and overt killing is another matter. First, separating societal permission to end a life from societal encouragement to do so is very difficult in practice. Of those who would choose to end life by deliberate and direct means, some will be heartrending cases that even now often occasion no substantial legal repercussions because all concerned agree that this is not what was really meant by the statutes against murder or assisting suicide. But many would undoubtedly be people who could have led personally rewarding lives, whose pain could have been assuaged, and whose deaths will be tragically premature. For some of these, death will occur largely because the society found it easier to allow an easy and private exit from the community, rather than to face the burden of adequately caring for and about people enduring great hardship. Permission to do a certain thing often inexorably leads to pressures for some persons to do that thing, perhaps especially when doing so is convenient for others. Consider that the availability of abortion and amniocentesis has undoubtedly led to pressures on at least some pregnant women to have Down's syndrome diagnosed and affected fetuses aborted.

Furthermore, neither dying nor medical decision making is the province of clear-sighted rational persons. Rather, the human beings who must face these choices are inevitably flawed, frail, and emotional. Dying people and those who care about them are quite commonly perplexed as to what one should do in such a situation. The availability of being killed may be attractive just to escape unaccustomed dependence, loss of control, or social isolation. In fact, insisting upon being killed may become the only way immediately available for the patient to maintain control, to rally support, and to prevent the uncertainty of outcomes from paralyzing the pursuit of other available goals. In this setting, encouraging and supporting the patient who might thereby be willing to persevere may become even more difficult if it were easy for all concerned to choose for the patient to be killed.

Perhaps public policies that would allow deliberate killings would yet be justifiable if very many people could thereby escape unmitigated and extreme suffering, while only a very few were placed at risk of a preemptorily shortened life. However, this is clearly not the case. There are at most very few persons with such severe and unrelievable suffering and there are very many whose lives and well-being would be endangered by the acceptance of their being killed. Although it is not clear that his pain could not be relieved, perhaps it could not be without thereby causing death. Then Dax would be forced to suffer for the protection of others. We do not commonly require one person to be a martyr and it is a decision that society should find troubling and in need of constant examination. But it is the best policy.

For the rare person who cannot find meaning or peace in the modes of existence that are available to him or her, we should be willing to provide the option of nearly continuous sedation. Continuous sedation is to be preferred to killing for two reasons. First, the patient is assured that those who provide care also value his or her life and are not willing to discard it lightly. Patients and potential patients are likely to find it quite disconcerting if the persons upon whom reliance must be placed in times of serious illness are also dispensers of quiet, publicly approved killings. Second, society is strengthened by a commitment to stand by the otherwise suffering person, a job that is difficult enough that it will be chosen on behalf of few patients. In effect, this will force care givers to be quite sure that no other option offers the patient more.

What would nearly continuous sedation have offered Dax? Certainly, at least after the first few weeks of electrolyte imbalance and respiratory troubles, continuous sedation would have been possible to achieve. It would, however, compromise the chances of medical success (both survival and functional ability) and the opportunities for self-determination. It still might have been a better option than abject nontreatment or abusive overtreatment. While it would be novel, the consent to long-term sedation could be fully valid if it held some safeguards, including provisions for periodic reevaluation and for decisions about likely complications.

If all of the foregoing had failed Dax and his situation was, in his own eyes, more miserable than being dead, what would happen to him if he had no assistance in suicide, but merely stopped his treatments? He would probably have been infected, had a period of a few days of increased discomfort, then become dehydrated and obtunded, and died. Should doctors have helped with this process? Surely, once his course of nontreatment was clear, Dax would have been dying and relieving his pain would be compassionate and appropriate and should not be considered the assisting of suicide. However, dying should not be hastened by some means that would seem to be direct killing, such as the giving of lethal doses of narcotics or nonmedical poisons.

Finally, it is all too easy to assume that care givers will be competent in law and ethics as well as medicine and nursing. As the film shows, this is certainly not the case. Ignorance and error are as difficult to eradicate as they are dangerous, and all the more so when what might be at stake is a life.

CONCLUSIONS

"New occasions teach new duties, time makes ancient good uncouth."[7] It has taken medical practice a generation to recognize that a new occasion is upon us—medical treatment can now convert most acute causes of death into chronic illnesses, and the treatment applied to chronic illness often largely shapes the nature and timing of death. What duties does this new occasion teach? It teaches the duty to provide for patients the dying that is "least bad" and the best possible living. No longer does the mandate to seek to extend life provide adequate guidance. In its stead, we must learn to serve the complex needs and desires of complex persons. But medical care providers should not accept the role of killers. We can and should relieve distress, sometimes at the cost of a briefer life. Yet, we must stay capable of cherishing those who are dependent, unpleasant, costly, severely disabled, or dying.

Dax Cowart should have been enabled to refuse treatment and die, but also he should have been respected and treated so as to make it as tolerable (even desirable) as possible to live. And irrespective of the outcome of these endeavors, health care providers should never be allowed directly and deliberately to kill him.

NOTES

1. *In re* Bertha Harris (D.C. Court of Appeals) 477 A. 2d, 724.

2. *People of California v. Barber and Nejdl,* Case No A 015586, Sup Ct. Los Angeles County, 1983.

3. President's Commission for the Study of Ethical Problems in Medicine and Biomedical and Behavioral Research, *Making Health Care Decisions* (Washington, D.C.: U.S. Government Printing Office, 1982).

4. President's Commission for the Study of Ethical Problems in Medicine and Biomedical and Behavioral Research, *Deciding to Forego Life-Sustaining Treatment* (Washington, D.C.: U.S. Government Printing Office, 1983), 34–36.

5. *Deciding to Forego Life-Sustaining Treatment,* 68–70.

6. Ibid., 87–89; Sacred Congregation for the Doctrine of the Faith, *Declaration on Euthanasia* (Vatican City, 1980).

7. James Russell Lowell, "Once to Every Man and Nation," *The Pilgrim Hymnal* (Boston: The Pilgrim Press, 1958).

Freedom vs. Best Interest:
A Conflict at the Roots of
Health Care 🜍
H. Tristram Engelhardt, Jr.

INTRODUCTION

DAX COWART SPEAKS ELOQUENTLY AS A PERSON
and through the film *Dax's Case*. Beyond the force of his personality, he commands our attention because of what he has endured
and because of the arguments he makes. He reminds us of the ways
in which individuals can heroically survive great suffering and can
fashion meaning for themselves. We have much to learn about the
virtues of courage and steadfastness in the face of suffering that
modern medicine cannot set aside. In this essay I will not explore
those issues but will instead address an important question Cowart
himself articulates. His arguments concerning personal liberties invite us to face a central conflict in ethics and the moral life: the conflict between respecting freedom and achieving the good.

Cowart and the film ask whether taking freedom seriously
means acknowledging the rights of competent individuals to dispose
of their lives in ways that others may judge imprudent. Freedom
can lead to tragic consequences that could have been avoided by
more paternalistic interventions. Because patients often regress
under the weight of pain and suffering and want and need to be
treated as children, medicine can properly intervene in paternalistic

79

fashions. The film raises the question of the limits of proper paternalism as Cowart presents himself as a competent individual who wants to be treated as his own master.

The conflict between freedom and best interests is not just a practical one, but a deeply philosophical one. The tension is at the heart of ethics and is most acute when freedom of choice is not endorsed simply because it is highly valued, but when it marks the limits of the authority of others to intervene. When such is the case, respect for the free choices of others depends on deontological or obligation- and rights-based moral considerations that cannot be reduced to interests in achieving particular goals and values. The obligation to respect the free choices of others when those choices do not involve force against the unconsenting innocent would then depend, to borrow a phrase from Robert Nozick, on freedom being a side-constraint, not an object of value.[1] Which is to say, freedom can make its claims on us even when most would hold that it causes more trouble than it is worth. In such circumstances, one will not be able to respect freedom without failing to realize very important values.

If there are restrictions on our moral authority to intervene in the peaceable free choices of others, then we may be morally constrained not to interfere coercively while they make choices we believe reasonable and prudent people would regret. We may also be constrained not to interfere coercively while individuals make choices we are sure they will in the future regret, were they able to survive and reassess the matter. The pathos of this tension can be appreciated by parents who have watched their grown children make tragic choices with profound consequences for their future lives. The children are free to do what they ought not to do. Respect for freedom and achievement of the good can collide.

The conflict between respecting the freedom of individuals and achieving their best interests has implications not just for ethical disputes among individuals. It lies as well at the core of a wide range of public disputes. The more individuals are allowed to choose freely, the more they harm their future selves and make the realization of social and political goals difficult. The resolution of this conflict will have profound implications regarding the moral authority of the state, not just for particular bioethical issues such as the right to refuse lifesaving treatment. If individuals have extensive freedoms over themselves, a whole range of state interventions to manage the lives of individuals will become morally problematic. Dax Cowart speaks to a quandary at the very core of ethics and public policy.

In this essay I will first outline the law and public policy that set the context for the film concerning Dax Cowart. My goal will be primarily to delineate the moral and philosophical assumptions that framed the difficulties he experienced. This analysis will also suggest reasons for being dubious about the moral right to impose treatment on unconsenting, competent individuals. Then I will look at the problem of whether to respect the present or future self when one has good reason to believe that an individual will in the future be grateful for having received treatment, even coercively imposed treatment. Does one honor a present request to end treatment or does one act to respect what one has good reason to believe will be the decision of the future self? Though a very philosophical question, it is one with intensely practical implications. But this is as one ought to expect: ideas, even abstract ideas, actually structure the ways in which we can and should live our lives. The work of the humanities in clarifying ideas is thus not distant from everyday action and public policy.

THE LAW, SUICIDE, AND TEXAS

It is ironic that Dax Cowart had difficulty in determining his own course of treatment in Texas, which in a number of ways has been distinguished by its original commitments to individual liberty. Texas, unlike all other common-law jurisdictions, never presumed that suicide was a crime, and until 1973 did not hold aiding and abetting suicide to be a crime. Prior to 1973, competent individuals probably could have successfully collected damages against others who interfered with their attempt to commit suicide. Nor would it have been a crime to aid and abet another's competent suicide. For instance, one could have put at the disposal of a severely burned individual the means to end life. In this, Texas law contrasted with the common-law tradition, which in general held that suicide and therefore aiding and abetting suicide were crimes. William Blackstone in his *Commentaries on the Laws of England* argued that, "[T]he suicide is guilty of a double offence; one spiritual, in invading the prerogative of the Almighty, and rushing into his immediate presence uncalled for; the other temporal, against the king, who hath an interest in the preservation of all his subjects."[2] Blackstone argued that the state existed to protect the rights of the deity. In a political system such as that of England, where the sovereign is also the head of the established church, such a position appeared more plausible than it would to us or to Englishmen today. However, this understanding has its descendants in the view that the state is the custodian of good public morals.

U.S. courts have continued to argue that the right to refuse treatment is limited. The court of the first instance in the Brophy case, which involved discontinuance of artificial hydration and nutrition, noted that: "There are circumstances in which the fundamental right to refuse extremely intrusive treatment must be subordinated to various State interests. Among the State interests which have been identified in prior cases: (1) the preservation of life; (2) the protection of the interests of innocent third parties; (3) the prevention of suicide; (4) maintaining the ethical integrity of the medical profession."[3] If the prevention of suicide itself is to be understood as a ground for intervening in the decision to refuse life-saving treatment by those who are not terminally ill, then suicide must be construed as an immoral act, against which the state has a right to protect itself or its citizens.[4] The last concern cited by the court, that of the integrity of the medical profession, is a general special interest in good public morals that could perhaps be defended in terms of its general utility. The first concern, that of the preservation of life, has deep roots in British law. Even before Blackstone had articulated the notion that the sovereign has a right in his subjects, Sir Edward Coke had articulated a similar position. In commenting on the case of the beggar Wright, who to increase his ability to elicit alms had a hand cut off, Coke noted that such was proscribed because "the life and members of every subject are under the safeguard and protection of the King . . . to the end that they may serve the King and their country, when occasion shall be offered."[5] Such an understanding of the relationship between citizens and the state presupposes what Robert Nozick has described in condemnation as "ownership of the people, by the people, and for the people."[6]

Such understandings of state authority contrast with the political sentiments of the Republic and the early State of Texas, which formed the background for the original Texas judicial approach to suicide and aiding and abetting suicide. In order to underscore their opinions regarding the limits of state authority, the constitution of the Republic and subsequent constitutions have endorsed what is tantamount to a right to revolution. "All political power is inherent in the people, and all free governments are founded on their authority, and instituted for their benefit; and they have at all times the inalienable right to alter their government in such manner as they think proper."[7] When Texas joined the United States, the last phrase was further developed in order to underscore this point. "[A]nd they have at all times the unalienable right to alter, reform, or abolish their form of government, in such manner as they may think expedient."[8] Texans joined this renunciation of the state as sacred or owning its citizens with a repudiation of the state as a protector of the rights of the deity or as divinely ordained by condemning both the priesthood and the military as "the eternal enemies of civil liberty, the ever ready minions of power, and the usual instruments of tyrants."[9]

This view of the state was in part drawn from Anglo-American understandings of democracy, which had moved with the frontier from Virginia to Texas. Individuals who participated in that migration tended to leave behind even the quasi-democratic view that the state gained its authority from some original or primordial contract through which founding individuals bound themselves and their descendants enduringly to the state. To them it was more plausible to see authority drawn from actual individuals. These assumptions were fortified by the anticlericism engendered in both Anglo- and Mexican-Texans by their experiences with an established church in Mexico.[10] As a result, the state was not seen to be endowed with divine right nor with the capacities to discern the best interests of its citizens better than individual citizens.

From a sociological point of view, this view of state authority could be expected. Men and women of the frontier tended to rely on themselves and stress individual capacities. In addition, given the inclinations and habits of life of many of the leading individuals who fashioned Texas, they were disinclined to see the state as having the authority to protect good public morals. Indeed, a great number of the founders of the Republic of Texas were individuals to whom the usual canons of civil probity were foreign.[11] The roots of this understanding of the state are even deeper than the foregoing suggest. They draw also from the political history that preceded the establishment of the Republic. The Republic of Texas came into existence after the failure of both the French and the Mexican Revolutions to bring lasting democracy and protection of individual rights. The idea that the state derived authority either from God or from a superior understanding of what was correct or proper conduct had been called into question. So, too, was the view of the state as the optimum custodian of the best interests of its citizens. Texas was the product of post-Enlightenment philosophical reflections and disappointments. To draw on a metaphor, the state as a successor to either Jerusalem or Athens had become untenable. When the Republic was founded, it drew on the pagan roots of Anglo-Saxon law, which saw the state as the creation of individuals and therefore as having limited authority.[12] It is thus not unexpected that, in the first days of the Republic, neither suicide nor dueling was a crime. If consent cured both theft and rape, it should render the consented-to taking of a life not a species of murder, but simply killing, an act about which the state can be neutral. Texas was unique among the

Anglo-American jurisdictions in not proscribing suicide, attempted suicide, or aiding and abetting suicide.

The implications of these views for Texas law on suicide were first articulated by the Texas Court of Criminal Appeals in 1902 when it held that, since suicide was not a crime, aiding and abetting suicide could not be a crime. The author of the Declaration of Independence of Texas, George Childress, had taken his life by stabbing himself in the stomach six times with a bowie knife, and the last president of Texas, Anson Jones, M.D., had taken his life after Texas became party to the U.S. Constitution. There was no evidence that suicide had been regarded as criminal. As a result, the court concluded, regardless of what "may have been the law in England, or whatever that law may be now with reference to suicides, and the punishment of persons connected with suicide, by furnishing the means or other agencies, it does not obtain in Texas." [13] In a subsequent case the Texas Court of Criminal Appeals drew a line between the authority of the secular state and the moral understandings of particular groups in opining that "it may be a violation of morals and ethics and reprehensible that a party may furnish another poison or pistols or guns or any other means or agency for the purpose of the suicide to take his own life, yet our law has not seen proper to punish such persons or such acts." [14] In short, Texas entered the twentieth century with an understanding of suicide and aiding and abetting suicide that was in many ways unique.

An abrupt realignment of Texas law concerning suicide and aiding or abetting suicide occurred in the early 1970s. In 1973 the legislature adopted the New Texas Penal Code, which now makes aiding suicide a felony. [15] Though this change in the law occurred without any evidence of abuse, [16] it did occur a year prior to Dax Cowart's tragic accident. From being an act without legal sanctions, aiding and abetting suicide in 1973 exposed the perpetrator to penalties ranging from two to ten years in prison and a fine ranging from $200 to $5000, depending on the circumstances. [17] Prior to the enactment of any living will and immediately subsequent to the change in Texas law, individuals might have concluded that patients had no legal and perhaps no moral right to refuse life-prolonging treatment.

Given the confused and evolving state of the law in Texas and other states, it is unclear the extent to which an individual such as Dax Cowart now has the legal right to refuse treatment, if competent and nonterminal. Living-will legislation has accented the right of individuals who are in a terminal state to refuse life-prolonging treatment. Contemporary legislatures and courts have generally taken less seriously than the old courts of Texas the claims of nonterminal, competent individuals that they have the right to end their lives by either action or omission. The claims of terminal patients to refuse treatment benefit from the fact that they can give little support to their dependents and the state can derive little from their services. Third parties have little to lose by respecting their requests. Still, in a recent case an appellate court in California, in reviewing the case of Elizabeth Bouvia, a severely handicapped woman suffering from cerebral palsy (but evidently neither pregnant nor with dependent minors), held that "a patient has the right to refuse any medical treatment or medical service, even when such treatment is labeled 'furnishing nourishment and hydration.' This right exists even if its exercise creates a 'life threatening condition.' . . . The right to refuse treatment is basic and fundamental." [18] In this holding California has taken a step toward the original position of the Texas courts. In fact, the concurring opinion in the April 16, 1986, decision went beyond the old Texas law and approached a policy of endorsing voluntary euthanasia.

> The right to die is an integral part of our right to control our own destinies so long as the rights of others are not affected. That right should, in my opinion, include the ability to enlist assistance from others, including the medical profession, in making death as painless and quick as possible.
>
> That ability should not be hampered by the state's

threat to impose penal sanctions on those who might be disposed to lend assistance.

The medical profession, freed of the threat of governmental or legal reprisal, would, I am sure, have no difficulty in accommodating an individual in Elizabeth's situation.[19]

The minority opinion suggested an approach that might have similarities with the policy of voluntary euthanasia currently proposed for the Kingdom of the Netherlands.[20] It also suggests legal and medical approaches quite different from those portrayed in the Dax Cowart film.

At stake is an understanding of state, communal, and professional authority that reaches back before the development of modern concepts of national sovereignty during the Renaissance. To what extent may a community, profession, or state force unconsenting innocent individuals to act in particular ways or to accept particular manipulations even when their actions and omissions do not involve unconsented-to force against others, and when they involve the collaboration of only consenting adults? Dax Cowart's case provides a particular example of this general issue. Under what circumstances may the state, physicians, or hospitals force patients to accept life-saving treatment?

The use of unconsented-to force presumably requires a justification. If that is the case, in order to have a moral warrant to employ coercive force against the unconsenting innocent, individuals or the state must at least show that: (1) the actions or omissions they endorse achieve what is correct or good to do, (2) they have the moral authority to realize what is correct or good to do without the consent of those involved, and (3) the use of coercive force will not do more harm than good. The first condition is particularly difficult to meet, given the collapse of the Enlightenment assumption that one can discover the morally authoritative ranking of goods and harms so as to judge how one ought to act in particular kinds of situations. For example, one will need to know which one ought to rank highest: liberty, prosperity, or security. If one gives first rank to liberty, it will become morally appropriate to forbid strong paternalistic interventions and to allow competent individuals to choose as they wish.[21] On the other hand, if one gives highest rank to personal security, then it may become appropriate to use coercive force to save even competent individuals from their imprudent choices. The difficulty is in choosing the correct ranking. Nor will it help to appeal to disinterested or ideal observers, for one will need to impute a moral sense to such observers in order for them to choose among different views of the good life, which incorporate different rankings of harms and benefits. The problem will then be how to choose the proper moral sense. Appealing to a higher moral sense will obviously not do, for one will need to continue to appeal to ever higher moral senses, ad infinitum.[22]

The more one is skeptical about the possibility of discovering the morally authoritative ranking of benefits and harms or of discovering what moral sense one ought to impute to impartial or disinterested observers, the more one will despair of grounding moral authority from an authoritative, rationally demonstrable understanding of the good life. If one cannot ground authority for coercive force in appeals to God, as with traditional British law, or simply appeal to force itself, then one must derive moral authority for coercive force from the consent of those involved.[23] Unless one credits some form of hereditary slavery through which one's ancestors irrevocably gave away one's freedoms over oneself in their consenting to one's government, then requests by individuals such as Dax Cowart to refuse life-prolonging treatment will constitute a bona fide withdrawal of authority from others to treat or intervene.

Rights to privacy, given this analysis, take on a new meaning. They indicate the limits of the plausible moral authority of others to intervene. If the authority of professions, communities, and states derives not from God nor from a rationally demonstrable authoritative view of the good life, then it must derive from the consent of those involved. Rights to privacy then signal where nonconsenting individuals have successfully withdrawn their authority from communal activities and from those who would interfere with their actions. To put matters in this way completely recasts the challenge Dax Cowart raised. It is not so much that competent individuals must justify their refusals of treatment. It is rather that others must justify their coercion of competent individuals who refuse treatment. Moral limits may still exist on the rights to refuse treatment because of dependent minors for whom there are continuing moral obligations. Moral limits may exist as well when one contracts to perform certain services, as for the armed forces. But still, the burden of proof shifts to the coercer. Those using coercive force must show that the prima facie right to dispose of one's self freely has been defeated—at least this shift in the burden of proof occurs insofar as serious doubts erode the traditional justifications for the use of coercive state or professional power.

The consequences for medical decision making within a secular pluralist society are thus more than sociological. They involve more than the difficulty of gaining the actual collaboration of numerous individuals with numerous views of the good life and the good death. There is, in addition, a better recognition of our inability intellectually to justify widely shared moral assumptions regarding the authority of professionals and the state. Which is to say, the pluralism allowed by the Enlightenment has in the end undercut the plausibility of many of the Enlightenment assumptions about the capacity of reason to discover a morally authoritative view of the good life. The more one examines the difficulty of gaining authority from conclusive philosophical arguments, the more one moves to gaining it from the consent of particular individuals. It is because of this that rights to privacy function as limits on the plausible authority of professions and the state. The answer to Dax Cowart's questions concerning the moral rights of others to interfere in the competent choices of individuals may thus become clearer, the more one looks at how one could possibly establish a moral warrant for such interventions. The more one looks, the more one is likely to embrace the original position of the state of Texas, which would have allowed competent individuals to make their own choices and suffer the consequences. Cowart's challenge is thus a radical one that leads not only to reassessing issues in bioethics and health care policy, but in public policy generally.

PRESENT AND FUTURE SELVES

Even if all of the foregoing seems plausible, one might ask which self one ought to respect. Through experience physicians find that there are groups of patients who initially want to reject all treatment, but who, if treated, generally are very grateful that their lives have been saved. The initial pain and suffering, one might contend, distort a patient's capacity to judge, even if the patient is not rendered incompetent. Beyond that, the patient who has been severely burned or rendered quadriplegic may not be able to envision future possibilities of a satisfactory life after rehabilitation. After rehabilitation, after exploring what life can be like despite serious handicaps, most of the patients will be glad that they were treated. Many who might be compelled to accept treatment might even be glad they were treated against their will. Which self ought one to respect: The present self, which will exist only for a short period of time if its wishes are respected and lifesaving treatment refused, or the future self, which will live a long and fulfilling life, albeit with major physical handicaps? Even if physicians would not see these considerations as providing them with the moral authority to coerce patients, they may at least make many physicians ambivalent about allowing a patient to die who could have been saved and rehabilitated. The discussions in *Dax's Case* concerning his rehabilitation illustrate this ambivalence.

It might seem that one way to solve the problem would simply be to total up the realization of the good, the enjoyment of pleasures, or the satisfaction of preferences over the full remaining likely scope of an individual's life in order to determine what ought to be done. If saving the person's life will likely lead to a positive balance, then the life should be saved. Such an approach would not only take freedom seriously, it would also presuppose something that does not appear to be available—an accurate way to measure the real value of goods achieved, pleasures enjoyed, or preferences satisfied. One needs an ideal observer with a univocal measuring rod, neither of which appears to be available to resolve the issue. For example, how intense would initial preferences not to be treated have to be in order to outweigh on the scale the satisfaction of preferences after re-habilitation is completed?

One might recall here an argument Dax Cowart already ar-ticulated about his experience in *Please Let Me Die*. Though he was willing to concede the possibility that rehabilitation might give him a life worth living, he was dubious that the pleasures and rewards of such a future life would outweigh the pains involved in realizing it. How could one ever know who was right? The future self might indeed forget the pains of the past self just as well as the past self might not be able to anticipate the rewards and pleasures of the fu-ture self. The measuring rods to compare pains, pleasures, and the satisfactions of preferences, insofar as they are available, change over time and between contexts. It is because of difficulties such as these, among others, that one is pushed back again to respect of freedom, not so much because one values it, but as a means of re-solving the controversy.

Still, one might attempt to resolve the controversy in favor of forcing treatment by making the following argument. Many be-lieve that a Ulysses contract is morally valid, that a past self can bind a future self. I may borrow money now, spend it and enjoy it, and promise to pay back the lender in the future. The present self gets the pleasure and the future self the debt. I can marry now or join the marines and create obligations for my future self. Or I might say to my crew, stuff your ears with cotton so that you do not get distracted by the Siren and bind me to the mast, and do not let me loose, no matter what I say. Why ought one to give greater weight to the past self's capacity to bind the future self when future selves often assert that they wish only that there had been someone forcibly to take their past selves in hand? Why do past selves count more than future selves?

One obvious response is that the present selves, not future selves, are all one has to deal with. A part of the collapse of the Enlightenment hope of reason justifying a concrete morally authoritative view of the good life is that individuals matter, if for no other reason than by default. Free and informed consent plays such a large role in medicine and public policy generally not simply because of a liberal commitment to highly valued freedom. It plays that role as a means of gaining authority for individual or communal action when no other plausible source is available. Real present persons can give real authority. Even past persons have a reality that is more secure than that of future persons—who may be, but who still may not. Past persons have created real debts and fashioned real obligations that can still bind those who are present. Future persons are but the possible objects of possible obligations. When they become present persons, they find themselves in a web of obligations fashioned by past persons.

To flesh out an answer here, one would have to ask another philosophical question. Should we be talking here about future and past selves or the past, present, and future of a self? Insofar as one has continuity through time, the matter is more clearly soluble. We are the kinds of beings who must choose for ourselves in the future. Insofar as we understand and appreciate the risks of those choices, we can commit ourselves for the future. If we are the source of authority, we will then have to be asked whether we are willing to make such choices. Others will have to judge whether we appear to be competent, whether we truly understand and appreciate the consequences of our actions. Even if our future selves stand to us somewhat as children do to their parents, it would be difficult to argue that we have an obligation to suffer great pain in order for them to come into existence. As future selves, they are not yet actual persons. Insofar as women may seek abortions on grounds of personal desire and social benefit, surely it would follow that individuals would be excused from bringing their future selves into existence at the cost of considerable pain and suffering. Still, there is the difficulty of deciding when and under what circumstances individuals competently refuse treatment.

As the film *Dax's Case* correctly suggests, this is a major problem in medicine. Patients in pain generally want to be left alone. Those in severe pain often would do almost anything to find surcease. This is not just an issue raised by severely burned or otherwise injured patients, but by pregnant women who as birth begins would do anything to have the issue brought to an end. Physicians over the centuries have reminded patients that, after a brief period of pain, they will be free of suffering and function will be restored. The principle that one must respect the freedom of competent individuals does not mean that one may morally acquiesce in incompetent decisions. Nor does the principle that one may not coerce mean that one may not peaceably manipulate. When a patient refuses lifesaving treatment, it is rarely morally appropriate simply to say that is fine, good-bye, and leave. Rather, it is usually obligatory to continue to attempt to make the acceptance of treatment the plausible choice. What is challenging about *Dax's Case* is precisely the fact that he is competent and well-informed. He presents us with the possibility of a patient who might very well competently refuse lifesaving treatment and be deaf to peaceable manipulations to reconsider the decision.

CONCLUSIONS

Dax's Case may very well lead us back to the previous Texas judicial approach to suicide and aiding and abetting suicide. We are attempting as a culture to learn to control powerful medical technologies that often succeed in preserving our lives only at the cost of a great deal of pain and suffering and at times with a quality of life we would not want to accept. Since human judgments regarding quality of life vary from person to person, and because the authority of others to intervene in the choices of competent individuals over their protests is dubious in most circumstances (other than, for example, when there may be dependent minors), we may have no other moral choice than to allow free individuals to choose for themselves. That was the old posture of Texas law. Competent individuals had to choose for themselves and take the consequences. This policy did not exclude civil commitment for the incompetent who were dangerous to themselves, nor should it exclude peaceable attempts to convince individuals to accept medical treatment, which in the future they will very likely be glad to have received. But since it is actual persons who make actual decisions, it is they who must be consulted. This is the point that Dax Cowart makes eloquently in the film. He would appear to be correct.

NOTES

1. Robert Nozick, *Anarchy, State, and Utopia* (New York: Basic Books, 1974), 30–34.

2. William Blackstone, *Commentaries on the Laws of England*, IV: 189.

3. *Brophy v. New England Sinai Hospital*, No. 85#0009-G1, (Mass. Trial Ct. Oct. 21, 1985), 39. This initial holding forbidding the discontinuation of artificial hydration and nutrition was reversed by the Massachusetts Supreme Judicial Court, on September 11, 1986.

4. Suicide in the strict sense must be understood to involve a direct intention to kill oneself by either omission or commission. One can intentionally effect acts of omission and commission, which may involve a near certainty of death, and which would not count as suicide because one's death was not directly intended, only foreseen. One can throw oneself on a hand grenade to save one's comrades, intending to absorb the shrapnel, while foreseeing the high likelihood of one's death (i.e., unless by happy fate the grenade is defective). One would not be intending one's death. It would not be an act of suicide. In this vein, moral theology has traditionally countenanced refusing life-saving treatment when it involved considerable pain, inconvenience, or cost, as long as one did not intend to die, only to avoid the pain, inconvenience, or cost involved in the treatment. See, for example, Daniel A. Cronin, *The Moral Law in Regard to the Ordinary and Extraordinary Means of Conserving Life* (Rome: Typis Pontificiae Universitatis Gregorianiae, 1958); Gerald Kelly, *Medico-Moral Problems* (St. Louis: Catholic Hospital Association, 1958); and Gerald Kelly, "The Duty of Using Artificial Means of Preserving Life," *Theological Studies* 11 (1950): 203–20.

5. Sir Edward Coke, *A Commentary Upon Littleton*, sec. 194.

6. Nozick, *Anarchy, State, and Utopia*, 290.

7. The Constitution of the Republic of Texas, March 17, 1836, Declaration of Rights, Second.

8. The Texas Constitution of August 28, 1845, Article I, Sec. 1.

9. The Texas Declaration of Independence, March 2, 1836.

10. Sister Paul of the Cross McGrath, "Political Nativism in Texas, 1825–1860" (Dissertation, Catholic University of America, 1930).

11. William R. Hogan, *The Texas Republic: A Social and Economic History* (Austin: University of Texas Press, 1980). Hogan quotes an entry from the diary of J. H. Henderson, who was in Houston on March 16, 1838, and who noted, "Had a serenade and much carousing—The Vice-Prest. Atty. Genl . . . & others arraigned for riotous conduct," 113. A letter from the times gives a similar insight: "So soon as I recovered from my serious illness I took a trip to Galveston Island with the President [Sam Houston] and the members of Congress, and saw *great* men in *high* life. If what I saw and heard were a fair representation, may God keep me from such scenes in the future. . . . On our return on Sunday afternoon, about one-half on board got mildly drunk and stripped themselves to their linens and pantaloons. Their Bacchanalian revels and blood-curdling profanity made the pleasure boat a floating hell. . . . I relapsed from the trip and was brought near to the valley of death." "Jottings from the Old Journal of Littleton Fowler," *Quarterly of the Texas State Historical Association*, 2 (July 1898): 82. This quote is also available in Hogan's study, 113–14.

12. Alongside the traditional cities of Jerusalem and Athens, with Jerusalem being the metaphor for the city founded on the authority of God and Athens the city founded on the authority of reason, one might put the old Texas capitol, Washington-on-the-Brazos as the city founded on mutual consent to the law as a means for resolving issues without recourse to unconsented-to-force. Washington-on-the-Brazos does not require the authority of God, nor does it require that reason be able to discover the concrete lineaments of good conduct. All it requires is the process of mutual consent and negotiation. As such, Washington-on-the Brazos is built on the ruins of the Enlightenment, though it has its ancestors in the roots of Anglo-Saxon common law and such pagan cities as Reykjavik.

13. *Grace v. the State*, 44 Tex. Crim. 193, 195 (1904); 69 S.W. Reporter 529, 530 (1902).

14. *Sanders v. State*, 54 Tex. Crim. 101, 105, 112 (1908); S.W. Reporter 68, 70 (1902).

15. Texas Penal Code Annotated, Sec. 22.08 (Vernon, 1974).

16. For a discussion of some of the aspects of the development of current

Texas law concerning suicide, see H. Tristram Engelhardt, Jr., and Michele Malloy, "Suicide and Assisting Suicide: A Critique of Legal Sanctions," *Southwestern Law Journal* 36 (November 1982): 1003–37.

17. See, for example, Texas Penal Code Annotated, Sec. 12.23 and 12.34.

18. *Bouvia v. L.A. Co. Sup. Ct.*, 2nd Civ. No. B019134 (April 16, 1986), 8f.

19. *Bouvia v. L.A. Co. Sup. Ct.* (J. Compton concurring), 2–3.

20. See Royal Netherlands Medical Association, "Standpunt inzake euthanasie," *Medisch Contact* 39 (1984). Also, the opinion by the Hoge Raad der Nederlanden, Strafkamer nr. 77.091, November 27, 1984.

21. By strong paternalism I mean to include interventions made on behalf of the best interests of an individual over that individual's protests. Paternalism on behalf of incompetents does not involve the violation of a competent contrary will. In fiduciary paternalism one acts on an explicit request of an individual or what one presumes would be that individual's competent wishes, were they known. Short-term, weak paternalistic interventions are usually examples of this last form of paternalism. See H. Tristram Engelhardt, Jr., *The Foundations of Bioethics* (New York: Oxford University Press, 1986), 279–84.

22. Ibid., 17–65.

23. Authority for coercive force can still be derived in a Kantian fashion from the implicit consent of all to a moral community. So, for example, all of those who reject the moral community cannot protest against coercive action, since they have rejected the basis of such a protest. Thus, all are authorized to come to the defense of individuals being killed or having their property transferred without their consent. Governments may also defend the agreed-to patterns of distribution of commonly owned properties. Engelhardt, *Foundations of Bioethics*, 71–74. One should note that Kant puts the matter in a slightly different way. See Immanuel Kant, *Metaphysik der Sitten* (Akademic Textausgabe), VI: 331–37.

Dax's Case: Implications for the Legal Profession 🦅
Patricia A. King

I FIRST LEARNED ABOUT DAX COWART'S TERRIBLE story in the mid-seventies from the videotape *Please Let Me Die*. Told in his own words and filtered through his pain, Dax's passionate plea to be allowed to die foreshadowed major legal and ethical issues concerning withholding or termination of treatment which were subsequently raised by the Quinlan and Bouvia cases among others.[1] Even today, law students who view the videotape are compelled to explore questions about the meaning of competence, the quality of life, and the deliberate hastening of death. Moreover, these students often experience powerful and unexplored emotions. For many of them, this viewing is their first significant confrontation with their own mortality or, perhaps worse, with the prospect of living indefinitely with some serious impairments produced by accident or disease.

While *Please Let Me Die* causes viewers to reflect deeply on matters of death and dying, it leaves many questions about Dax and his situation unanswered. First, it does not tell the viewer what happened to Dax after his filmed interview with Dr. Robert White, the psychiatrist who had been engaged to evaluate his mental competency. Second, it does not explore the legal and ethical dilemmas posed for others who alone were in a position to help Dax achieve his wish to die. One of the most gripping features of Dax's plight was his utter helplessness. He not only was unable to leave the hospital by himself but he also was unable to summon outside assistance by himself. In order to die quickly and painlessly, he was totally dependent upon the help of others. Consequently, although *Please Let Me Die* presents Dax's perspective on his situation in a memorable way, it introduces viewers only by implication to the broader legal and ethical issues generated by Dax's remarkable circumstances.

For these reasons, I was curious to see the film *Dax's Case* because I hoped it would fill out more of the details and explore some of the issues not treated in *Please Let Me Die*. Happily, *Dax's Case* does exactly that. Not only do we learn about Dax's life after his release from the hospital, but the new film explores as well the issues that Dax's plea to die posed for his family, his friends, and those who cared for him. It places Dax at the hub of a series of relationships—with his mother, his lawyer, his friends, his nurses, and his physicians—and thereby broadens and enriches our understanding of the interactions of professionals and family members with a person who wants to die. By drawing our attention to this web of interactive relationships in which the conduct of one affects all, *Dax's Case* pushes us to reflect further on the nature of obligations, legal and ethical, potentially generated by such relationships. Moreover, it gives us a glimpse of the impact of decisions made in this context on the broader society. In short, *Dax's Case* makes clear that an individual's decision to die may involve more than questions of individual rights and autonomy, even though as a practical and legal matter it might be necessary to resolve disputes among persons in conflictive relationships by an appeal to a concept of individual rights and autonomy.

I

As a lawyer and a law teacher, I had been particularly intrigued by a statement that Dax had made in *Please Let Me Die*. In response to a question from Dr. White about what steps he was taking to get out of the hospital, Dax replied: "Well, right now I'm trying to exhaust every legal means that I can find. And I'm working through attorneys and so far I haven't had much luck, it's something that I found out attorneys, at least ethical ones, don't want to touch, probably for fear of getting bad publicity."[2] I had always wondered why Dax could not persuade a lawyer to help him obtain a court order releasing him from the hospital. Dax had a potentially significant personal injury suit as a result of the gas explosion that burned him. It therefore was likely that a lawyer had been retained to handle Dax's personal injury suit. If Dax did have a lawyer, why had that lawyer not responded to Dax's pleas for legal assistance by bringing the matter to the attention of an appropriate court? Did that lawyer have an obligation to respond personally to such a plea or at least to find some other lawyer who might? While Dax's caretakers and other friends might have been concerned about the moral and legal implications of "helping him to commit suicide," a lawyer could easily have sought resolution of the legal aspects of the dilemma created by Dax's pleas by bringing the matter to the attention of a court.

On viewing *Dax's Case*, I learned that Dax did have a lawyer. Rex Houston, who regarded the entire Cowart family as his clients and his friends, represented both Dax and his mother in their personal injury litigation against the owners of the pipeline which caused the explosion that injured Dax and killed his father. But Houston was never willing to help Dax obtain court authorization for the termination of his treatment or for his release from the hospital. Indeed, he apparently worked to circumvent Dax's desires to die at every stage of his treatment.

In *Dax's Case*, Houston recounts that he began an immediate investigation of the accident in order to file a lawsuit as soon as possible. He knew that he needed to get to trial quickly. Since Dax was single and without dependents, his lawsuit would not be worth very much if he were to die. As a living plaintiff, however, Dax had a very valuable lawsuit. If Dax were still alive at the conclusion of the legal proceedings, Houston stood to recover a large sum of money which would be available either for Dax's future or for the benefit of his heirs. Eventually he was able to settle out of court and to establish a substantial financial trust for Dax.

Moreover, as *Dax's Case* makes clear, Houston's concern extended beyond being responsible for the Cowart lawsuits. He was readily available to the family during Dax's extended stay in the hospital. Physicians at all three hospitals where Dax received treatment recall that Houston played an important role along with Dax's mother in reaching treatment decisions with medical personnel during periods when Dax was protesting his wish to die. Houston continued to be available to Dax after he was released from the hospital. He encouraged and counseled Dax about the future and helped him gain admission to law school. He even attended to such details as persuading Dax's mother to allow him to drink beer at home despite her religious objections to having alcohol in the house.

The picture that emerges from *Dax's Case* suggests that Houston played multiple roles. These multiple roles make it especially difficult to sort out the nature and scope of his legal obligations to Dax. It might be useful before exploring those roles more closely to outline Houston's involvement with Dax during his fourteen months of treatment at three different facilities. While Dax was at Parkland Hospital from July 24, 1973 until March 12, 1974, Houston represented Dax and his mother in their lawsuits against the pipeline company which caused the explosion that injured Dax and killed his father. These lawsuits were pursued simultaneously (I do not know whether the suits were filed jointly or separately) during a period in which Dax regularly expressed a desire to die and at a time when he may have been at odds with his mother, who was signing the consent forms for his treatment. But there is no evidence that Dax ever explicitly refused treatment or sought legal assistance to gain discharge from the hospital during his stay at Parkland Hospital.[3] Nor is there any evidence that Houston represented Dax in any professional capacity during the last month at Parkland Hospital after the lawsuit was settled in February 1974.[4]

From March 12, 1974 to April 15, 1974, Dax was treated at

the Texas Institute for Research and Rehabilitation. It was during this period that Dax for the first time refused treatment. When his condition became critical as a result of his refusing treatment, Houston and Mrs. Cowart were summoned to talk with him about resuming treatment. Subsequently, a decision was made to transfer Dax to a hospital with a burn ward where he could be treated properly. Apparently Houston did not act in any official capacity during this period. Rather he served as a family advisor and friend.[5]

On April 15, 1974, Dax was transferred to John Sealy Hospital at the University of Texas Medical Branch at Galveston. There is evidence that during this period Houston explicitly refused to have any part in Dax's efforts to refuse treatment or to secure legal assistance in gaining release from the hospital. In a background interview for the film, Houston said: "I told Donnie (Dax) that I could get him out of the hospital any time, but then what? Was his mother going to have to take care of him while he died a slow death? I told him that if he stayed in the man's hospital, you got to do what the man says."[6] Houston also reported that he had "warned Cowart (Dax) about trying to find some 'jake-legged' lawyer to represent him because no reputable lawyer would get involved in such a case."[7]

In watching both *Please Let Me Die* and *Dax's Case* and in reviewing additional material about Houston's role, one cannot avoid being caught up in the vortex of emotion, pain, and suffering endured by Dax and those who took care of him or made decisions about his future. While Houston's conduct comes through as extraordinarily paternalistic, I have no doubt that he and all the other participants acted in good faith and did what they thought was best in the midst of a human tragedy that extended over many months. Thus, I do not want what I write here to be in any way viewed as a condemnation of Houston's conduct—conduct, it should be noted, that occurred many years before there was any legal consensus on whether a competent person could terminate treatment. Rather, it is my purpose to use what I know about the facts of Houston's role in Dax's case to raises questions for lawyers about the nature and extent of their obligation should they find themselves in similar circumstances today.

II

Houston was in a very difficult position. He represented Dax and his mother. Adequate representation of both depended, however, on mother and son having the same or significantly similar interests. To the extent that the relationship between Dax and his mother became antagonistic and their interests diverged, Houston could not adequately have represented them both.

Houston's situation was further complicated because he represented Dax and his mother in their personal injury suits at a time when Dax was regularly expressing the desire to die. The fact that Dax repeatedly expressed a wish to die created several problems, perhaps even conflicts of interest, for Houston. First, Dax's desire to die was at odds with the strategy of the lawsuit that Houston was pursuing on Dax's behalf—to maximize the monetary potential of Dax's lawsuit, which would happen only if Dax lived. Second, to the extent that Houston's fee was dependent upon the size of any ultimate recovery for Dax's injuries, his own interests were in direct conflict with his client's interests. Finally, Dax's wish to die raised the possibility that Dax's interests were in conflict with the interests of his mother. She was recently a widow who was trying to cope with the fact that her oldest son wished to die. If we assume that Dax was legally competent, she should have played no role in decisions concerning his care. Yet that clearly was not the case. She was always consulted about treatment decisions and, at least during his stay at Parkland Hospital, signed the necessary forms for his care, perhaps in conflict with Dax's requests.

Assuming that Dax was competent, it would appear that minimally Houston should have disclosed to Dax the facts of his situation and the possible conflicts of interest. Dax might have decided to pursue his treatment. Alternatively, if Dax still wanted to terminate his treatment, he had several options. Dax might have decided to end the dual representation. He might have decided to settle the lawsuit at that point or asked for an expedited trial if that were possible. Houston could also have made his own decision about whether he wanted to, or indeed could, continue as Dax's lawyer. The record is silent on whether Houston actually made such disclosures to Dax. Whether he did or did not is unimportant at this point. What is significant is to examine the powerful countervailing forces that might have led Houston or others in similar circumstances to avoid discussing these matters with the client.

Houston's already difficult position was further complicated by the fact that he not only represented Dax and his mother, but he was also a friend to both Dax and his mother. There is surely nothing inherently inappropriate about a lawyer representing a friend although many lawyers avoid representing relatives or close friends. Indeed, in a well-known piece, "The Lawyer As Friend: The Moral Foundations of the Lawyer-Client Relation," Charles Fried analogizes the lawyer's role to that of friend.[8] Playing the role of both lawyer and friend is always fraught with problems, however, and friendship might increase the chances that a lawyer will fail to disclose to the client/friend.

The problem is that a lawyer who is also a friend often exercises more power and authority in a relationship than a person who is only a friend would be able to exercise. Charles Fried recognized, although he did not analyze, the problems generated by the overlap in roles. He wrote: "Analogizing the lawyer to a friend raises a range of problems. . . . These have to do with the lawyer's benevolent and sometimes not so benevolent tyranny over and imposition on his client, seemingly authorized by the claim to be acting in the client's interests. Domineering paternalism is not a normal characteristic of friendship."[9] This enhanced authority of a person who is both lawyer and friend is surely illustrated in Dax's case.

"Domineering paternalism" is not the only potentially adverse consequence of mixing the role of lawyer and friend. Often a person playing both roles exerts extraordinary authority and influence over others as well. A professional view of a situation can disarm defenses that might be raised against mere individual views and can lay claim to acceptance by third parties regardless of the client's own personal views. For example, as noted earlier, Rex Houston became an important decision maker with the doctors during their difficult periods with Dax. Undoubtedly Houston's support was reassuring in view of possible legal consequences that might have flowed from their decision to continue to treat Dax over his objection. A friend who is only a friend probably would not have been able to exert such influence. The presence of this friend/lawyer relationship, therefore, further complicates what is already a tough problem: namely, the nature and extent of a lawyer's obligations in circumstances similar to those of Dax's case. It is incumbent, therefore, upon a lawyer wearing the hats of both friend and lawyer to keep separate the roles both for the lawyer's own sake and for the sake of others with whom the lawyer deals.

Doubts about a client's capacity to make a sound decision—especially when the client is also a friend—are used often to justify decisions not to disclose. Perhaps the "domineering paternalism" of all those who came in contact with Dax, including Dax's lawyer, resulted from their belief that Dax, despite his obviously rational and articulate pleas, was not really able to make sound decisions. Dax after all had endured long and painful traumas, and he was undoubtedly depressed. Yet the mere belief that a client is incapable of making a wise decision cannot alone justify continued disregard of the client's pleas. Moreover, even incompetent persons have interests, and those interests in some circumstances are clearly separate and distinct from the interests of those individuals on whom society normally relies to provide for such persons. Indeed, in Dax's case, as I mentioned above, his interests were possibly in conflict with those of his mother.

At some point, therefore, the incompetency issue must be resolved by neutral deciders. Lawyers are in an especially good position to bring about that process. While impartial and unbiased legal representation might in some circumstances be helpful, lawyers must be cautious in such representation. The lawyer is clearly charged with acting in the client's best interests, but what does that entail when the client is not competent? Because incompetent persons are incapable of speaking for themselves, it is impossible for an advocate to be sure what those interests are. It is impossible, therefore, to know whether the lawyer is really responsive to the client's needs or is simply asserting his or her own values. If Dax's competency was in doubt, an attorney might have attempted to have Dax's views placed before some institution with the power to make definitive decisions about his competency and about the conflict between Dax and others in charge of his treatment.

Since an attorney cannot be a truly effective advocate in the absence of a client capable of articulating his or her own interests, some writers have urged that legal representatives of incompetent clients play some role other than that of advocate. A legal representative could play the role of fact finder and thereby assist some independent body to make decisions about an incompetent person's interests. A lawyer who was a fact finder might have thoroughly investigated Dax's situation and reported the findings to a neutral decision maker. However the lawyer's role is regarded—as advocate or fact finder—one inevitably reaches the conclusion that the final decision should be made by a neutral body. The recognition that some issues should be resolved in another forum is not a plea for judicial resolution of all problems that arise in the medical treatment of incompetent persons. It is, however, a recognition of the need to consider the procedural as well as the substantive aspects of dilemmas raised by the care of incompetent patients where there are actual or perceived differences about appropriate care. Surely haphazardly allowing those who happen to be in attendance to decide will not suffice.

Perhaps the crux of Dax's situation is that all of those in a relationship with him—his mother, his doctors, and his lawyer—exceeded the boundaries of their relationships with him. All failed to realize the limitations of their roles—of their special areas of expertise. Dax's pleas raised issues outside of parental, medical, or legal expertise. Since lawyers are trained to appreciate the importance of procedural fairness, perhaps they should be especially alert to the plight of persons like Dax. Indeed, the traditional understanding of the lawyer's role suggests that a lawyer in such circumstances should try to accomplish the client's objectives. And in the rare instance where a lawyer believes that he or she cannot in good conscience carry out the client's wishes, the lawyer should put the client in contact with a lawyer who does not have such reservations.

III

If we assume that Dax was competent to make decisions for himself, then the "domineering paternalism" of those who were in a relationship with him is hard to justify. Perhaps there is more to the "domineering paternalism" at work in Dax's case than may appear from just an understanding of the facts of that particular case. I would suggest that such paternalism may be related to the inherent nature of the lawyer-client relationship itself.

Legal ethics—concern for the philosophical and ethical premises of legal professionalism as opposed to concern for adherence to a professionally promulgated code of ethics—is still in the early stages of theoretical development. The intensified interest in this subject is primarily a post-Watergate phenomenon because the unraveling of that scandal revealed the heavy involvement of lawyers. Recognition of moral and ethical dilemmas of the kind faced by Rex Houston is of recent origin. In part the concern is relatively new because the concept of professions, of which law is only one, is itself a nineteenth-century development. The philosophical subject of professional ethics has really only come into existence in the last few decades. Moreover, it was medicine, not law, that was the first of the professions to capture theological, philosophical, and public attention. Beginning in large measure with revelations at the Nuremberg trials of physician participation in unethical experiments on human beings, the concern for medical ethics accelerated in recent decades to cover areas like abortion, euthanasia, and allocation of scarce medical resources, in addition to research with human subjects.

Moreover, much of the budding theoretical literature of legal ethics is not concerned with Houston's dilemma. Instead attention is often focused on the overarching issue of the limitations of the traditional understanding of the lawyer's role as opposed to some alternative models which have in common greater concern for collective or societal rather than individual interests. The traditional understanding of the lawyer's role emphasizes that the lawyer owes the client absolute loyalty and fidelity. The lawyer's role is to advance the client's interest to the limits of professional ethics. Moreover, the lawyer is to remain detached and aloof from the client. In that way the lawyer's personal belief system is not allowed to interfere with the accomplishment of the client's goals and objectives. The traditional understanding of the lawyer's role then is grounded in appeal to the autonomy, individuality, responsibility, and dignity of the client. The lawyer's function is to enhance the autonomy of the client. This devotion to the client's needs consequently precludes consideration in most instances of the needs of others or of society in general.

In our society the lawyer has a formal and practical monopoly over access to authoritative dispute resolution institutions. Lay persons such as Dax need access to such institutions to learn what rights they have as well as to enforce rights already recognized. In this respect access to such institutions is a prerequisite to full participation in this society. The lawyer in providing practical access makes it possible for the client to function more effectively. In one respect Dax was very fortunate. He at least had a lawyer.

Ironically, however, this value of enhancing client autonomy is subverted—as arguably it was in Dax's case—by practices and attitudes of legal professionals.[10] The relationship between lawyer and client is inherently unbalanced. And this inherent inequality in my view subverts the goal of enhancing client autonomy. The inherent inequality, I believe, is characteristic of all professions and is at the heart of any professional relationship. Because the legal professional is gatekeeper to much of what is of value in society, the inequality has particularly pernicious effects.

Lawyers are commonly regarded as being members of an elite

occupation called a profession. For purposes of this discussion let me state four characteristics that are commonly regarded as distinguishing professions from other occupations.[11] First, persons in order to be considered members of a profession are required to undergo a prolonged period of training in a body of abstract and specialized knowledge. Second, a profession is granted the right by society to control its own conduct. It is self-regulating and determines who can legitimately do its work and how that work should be done. Third, professionals have direct, continuous relationships with lay persons whom they assist. Fourth, professional activities are regarded as being particularly useful and productive for such lay persons and for society. In the case of law, a lawyer's special competence is to act as an advisor or counselor and, if need be, a litigator in order to help lay persons realize objectives and goals permitted by law but not obtainable without a lawyer's special competence. These four characteristics of a profession are what generates the imbalance between the professional and the client.

These lawyer-professionals have thus been endowed by society and often by their clients with special expertise and status. The "specialness" is reinforced by a lawyer's education and training. Lawyers have a special language and access to mysterious processes. Lawyers generally think they are entitled to feel aggrieved when clients decline to follow their advice. Not surprisingly, lawyers come to see themselves as superior to and wiser than their clients. Lawyers believe they should make decisions because they have superior skills and knowledge. And if the client does not follow the advice, "By God he had better get another lawyer," is the extreme way I heard one attorney put it.

The consequence of professional self-regulation is that lawyers are likely to see themselves as accountable to peers rather than clients. For example, it is a matter of some debate about whether lay persons can serve as part of the attorney disciplinary process. There are few ways in which lawyers may be held accountable to clients. Even the ability to withhold a fee is seldom enough to overcome the lawyer's mystique or to hold the lawyer accountable to the client.

Not only is a lawyer likely to look to peers rather than clients as a point of reference, but the vulnerability of the client mitigates against a lawyer using a client's judgment to check himself or herself. A lawyer's special competence is to help persons realize objectives that could not be achieved without a lawyer's special knowledge and skill; consequently, a lawyer is unlikely to take seriously the views and wishes of a less informed lay person. This tendency is reinforced where the lawyer believes that the client's judgment is colored by being too closely involved in the matter at hand—that the client lacks objectivity. Moreover, since the client's own conduct often contributes to the creation of the problem, it is easy to argue that the client is too involved to make rational decisions.

Perhaps the biggest problem generated by the inherent inequality in the professional client role is the fact that by training and socialization a professional tends to focus only on that part of the client's life that comes within the attorney's special expertise. Rex Houston was confident about proceeding with the personal injury suit and the importance of acting quickly. He was in an area that he knew well, and he was confident that he was doing the right thing. He assumed that Dax would feel the same. Yet a focus on the client that involves only the professional's area of expertise risks treating the client as a mere one-dimensional object. Houston by education and training was not prepared to comprehend fully the impact of living in great pain, with a radically different lifestyle. It would have been hard for a lawyer to appreciate the impact on Dax of something as common as the reactions of others to his disfigurement. Moreover, extracting monetary payment from a person or an institution who has caused harm is not always the primary motivation of those who are in need of a lawyer's skills. The law of domestic relations presents many issues of this kind. For example, a person in the process of obtaining a divorce may not wish to extract all that the law will allow if doing so will entail the loss of something more important—such as continued good relations with the other parent of one's children.

One could argue that Dax was in no danger of being treated

like an object because there was an abundance of concern for him as a son, friend, etc. But as I indicated before, familiarity with one's client does not necessarily promote respect for the person. The fact of a friendship coupled with a professional relationship may indeed increase paternalism by giving the person who is friend additional ways of imposing his or her own values and wishes.

If the lawyer/client relationship is an inherently unequal relationship which subverts client autonomy, what can be done to create more balance—to put the client in control? There are surely many possible approaches: simplify legal language, alter processes and access to institutions, modify legal education and training, and so on. These approaches would require, however, years of institutional reform before they would be useful. One approach could be borrowed and modified from medical ethics for use in the lawyer-client relationship. That approach is to make the concept of informed consent a central aspect of the lawyer-client relationship. Although the traditional understanding of the lawyer's role purports to enhance autonomy and respect for persons, that understanding has never had at its core an appreciation of the value of informed consent in achieving that goal. Ironically, this ethical and legal obligation has been established for physicians in large measure by the efforts of lawyers who have not bothered to impose the concept, either ethically or legally in many cases, on themselves.

Historically lawyers were not subject to the same constraints as physicians because the concept of consent to professional intervention was lodged in the law of battery which sought to protect bodily integrity. Lawyers rarely, if at all, need to touch their clients; therefore, the law of battery did not act as a constraint on their activities. As a matter of tort law, however, a physician could not intentionally touch the body of another without obtaining the other's permission. Even if the physician performed an operation that provided a benefit to the patient, the physician committed a battery if the physician did not first obtain the patient's consent (though damages were often reduced in such cases). The importance of having a point beyond which it is risky for the professional to proceed is underscored by the facts of Dax's treatment as presented in *Dax's Case*. It is apparent that Dr. White was called in as a consultant because Dax refused to give consent to skin graft surgery and the doctors were afraid to proceed in the absence of such consent. But for the legal requirement that the doctors were afraid to ignore, Dax might have been treated over his objection for an indefinite period of time.

There is a growing acceptance of the view, however, that a theory of informed consent grounded in the concept of battery is too limited. If the autonomy of the individual is to be accorded significant legal recognition, then a theory of informed consent must be grounded not so much in the need to protect bodily integrity as in the need to emphasize human dignity and the right of the individual to control his or her conduct. This latter approach to a theory of informed consent is particularly important if one is to apply the concept to the lawyer-client relationship.

Establishing the contours of a theory of informed consent for lawyers is clearly beyond the scope of this essay. But if it is to enhance dignity and to give control to clients, any such theory must take into account a particular need for assent and adequate disclosure. For example, a lawyer often acts, purportedly in the best interests of the client, without even discussing alternative courses of action with the client. Often the client has a particular objective in mind, such as obtaining a divorce, but there is little or no discussion between attorney and client of the means to be employed in attaining that end. As a result, the client does not actually give consent to many of the intermediate decisions made in a case.

Not only is the agreement aspect of informed consent important in thinking about applying the concept to lawyers, but the issue of agreement is inextricably linked to the issue of adequate disclosure. If anything, the issue of what is adequate disclosure is more complex in law than in medicine because there is no commonly accepted endpoint in law. At least in medicine, most persons want to be restored to health and well-being or as close to that state as is possible. As *Dax's Case* illustrates, however, this is not so clear even in medicine. Yet I believe the generalization holds in comparing medicine with law. For example, in procuring a divorce, the client's primary motive might be revenge, harassment, a good long-term relationship, peace of mind, expiating guilt, or all of the above. The ethical lawyer cannot assume that in a given situation one or more of these goals is the one sought by the client. People in reality are very complex. Individual goals are set in a social context in which individual fulfillment depends on many things including relationships with others. How legal proceedings might influence relations with a person's family, friends, finances, or even a person's freedom is important information for the client that strongly influences what might be the best course of action for the client. It is critical that lawyers share information with their clients if the clients' and not the lawyers' values are to predominate.

I have not attempted to exhaust the considerations that should be developed in applying a concept of informed consent to the lawyer-client relationship, but I have emphasized those elements—actual agreement and adequate disclosure—that I believe to be the most important. I also believe that the absence of informed consent played a major role in the decision making for Dax. For example, I doubt that Dax would have consented to his lawyer cooperating with his physicians in continuing his treatment. Prolonged interaction between Dax and his lawyer, undertaken with the value that the client's wishes were paramount and that the lawyer should not proceed without explicit authority from the client, might have brought about a different result. Dax's lawyer was the one person who could have provided Dax with what he wanted—access to a court with the authority to allow Dax to terminate his treatment if it believed that such a decision was warranted under the law. I do not mean to suggest by stressing client autonomy and the means for enhancing that autonomy that a professional's obligation to the client should take precedence over the ethical and religious concerns of the professional involved. The obligation of the professional to the client would seem to require, however, that the professional attempt to find a willing lawyer as an alternative to abandonment.

Finally, it should come as no surprise that *Dax's Case* reveals that Dax wanted to attend law school after his release from the hospital. As he wrote some years later, "If there exists any such thing as self-evident or naturally endowed rights, the right to control over one's own body must surely be among them."[12] Perhaps Dax believed that by becoming a lawyer he could unravel the process by which our systems of law and ethics had cost him the right to control his own life.

NOTES

1. *In re* Quinlan, 70 N.J. 10, 355 A.2nd 647, cert. denied, 429 U.S. 922 (1976); *Bouvia v. Superior Court of Los Angeles County*, 179 Cal. App.3d 1127, 225 Cal.Rptr.297 (Ct. App. 1986). The California Supreme Court refused to hear an appeal of the appellate ruling.

2. "Please Let Me Die" (transcript of videotape) in *Law, Science and Medicine*, Judith Areen et. al. (Mineola, N.Y.: Foundation Press, 1984), 115.

3. Kliever, Lonnie D. Letter to the author, 12 February 1988.

4. Ibid.

5. Ibid.

6. Ibid.

7. Ibid.'

8. Charles Fried, "The Lawyer as Friend: The Moral Foundations of the Lawyer-Client Relationship," *Yale Law Review* 85 (1976): 1060.

9. Ibid., 1066.

10. For an excellent discussion of the nature of the relationship between lawyer and client to which this author is indebted, see Richard A. Wasserstrom, "Lawyers as Professionals: Some Moral Issues," *Human Rights* 5 (1975): 15–24.

11. See Areen, *Law, Science and Medicine*, 259.

12. Ibid., 1117.

Taken to the Limits: Pain, Identity, and Self-Transformation 🩺
William J. Winslade

DAX'S CASE IS A VISUAL AND VERBAL COLLAGE THAT provides glimpses of a rich and subtle drama about pain, identity, and self-transformation, reveals a multiplicity of interpersonal values and value conflicts, and offers insights about the meaning of life and death. It is extraordinary because it captures, through carefully juxtaposed interviews and images, more than a decade of a personal and family tragedy, pain, conflict, and understanding as well as misunderstanding. In this essay I attempt to unravel as well as interweave themes about personhood, values, and meaning. I try to show how changes in personal identity are symbolized by the change of name from Donald Herbert "Donnie" Cowart to Dax Cowart. Changes in the meaning of Dax's life are manifested in his desire to die, to refuse treatment, or to commit suicide. Although Dax has undergone a significant loss of bodily and physical capacities, he has also undergone a self-transformation that the name change partially signifies.

WHO IS DAX COWART?

After the propane gas explosion, Donald Herbert "Donnie" Cowart ran through the fire hollering for help. When a nearby farmer arrived, he asked for a gun and told the farmer, "Can't you see I'm a dead man? I'm going to die anyway." Despite his prediction and his plea, he did not die. And yet he did. The charred and disfigured body and sightless eyes were no longer Donald "Donnie" Cowart, the handsome young athlete, pilot, and rodeo rider. Art Rousseau, a friend briefly interviewed in *Dax's Case,* made the insightful remark that there was not going to be Don Cowart anymore. Rousseau was right, at least in part.

In the interviews with Dr. Duane Larson as well as Dax's mother, it is interesting that they always refer to Dax as "Don" or "Donnie." Rex Houston, Dax's attorney, sometimes calls him Dax and sometimes refers to him as "Don" or "Cowart." Dr. Robert White, the psychiatrist, more formally but precisely speaks of "Mr. Cowart." Does it matter what name is used? After all, we know whom they are referring to. Or do we?

Although no explanation is given in the film of *Dax's Case,* Dax has told me and others that he changed his name from Don, Donnie, or Donald to Dax because he wanted to know for sure when people were talking to him.[1] Partly because of his hearing loss, and partly because of his blindness, he has trouble knowing when he is being specifically addressed. I don't doubt that this is a true and a sufficient explanation for the name change.[2] Whatever reason Dax may have had for changing his name, it is also possible to view it as a sign of a modification, though not a total loss, of his personal identity. The following interpretation may help us better understand the answer to the question, "Who is Dax Cowart?"

The nature of personal identity has perplexed philosophers for centuries. Are persons only their bodies? Only their minds? Or are they some mysterious union of mind and body? Dax suffered deep third-degree burns over 65 percent of his body that seriously damaged both eyes, both ears, and both hands. The familiar, recognizable body of Donald Cowart was virtually destroyed. He lost not only his sight, hands, and partial hearing capacity, but also part of his identity.

His body had served him well in his physical adventures as a youth and instinctively drove him as he ran from the explosion and fire that engulfed him. Almost immediately thereafter his body became a locus of excruciating and unspeakable pain. It was the relentless, tortuous pain and loss of physical function that Dax realized would extinguish his independence and freedom. He knew he would be extremely dependent on others; he comments about how his dependence on others extended to even his most private needs. He had lost much of his body, been robbed of his capacities to care for himself, and been disfigured beyond recognition. Dax realistically observes that at least he doesn't have to endure the stares of others. His blindness mercifully protects him.

In contrast to the loss of his body, the mind of Don Cowart remained remarkably intact. Even in his conversation with the farmer about the gun, one glimpses the decisive and logical thinking that characterizes Don as well as Dax. In the videotape *Please Let Me Die* made less than a year after the explosion and in the later interviews in *Dax's Case*, Dax always appears lucid and logical. In brief personal contacts with Dax in 1983 and again in 1986, my impression was reinforced. Dax not only displays clarity of thought, but also tenacious beliefs and a powerful independence of will. His mother remarks that "Donnie" had always been "very independent." This, I suspect, is a Texas-sized understatement.

This is not to deny that Dax experienced periods of depression and despair—as he readily reports. It is not to deny that during his tankings he felt abused and dreamed that he was a victim of sadistic torture. Dax felt bored, helpless, suicidal, angry, frustrated, and undoubtedly many other dark sensations, feelings, emotions, and moods. But what he retained throughout, apparently, was the ability to think—to think clearly, logically, and coherently in spite of the pain, blindness, and total dependence on others. His body was devastated but his mind was intact. Robert Burt argues in *Taking Care of Strangers* that his clarity of thought and strength of will about wanting to die were so definitive and final that one supposes they were defensive and concealed underlying ambivalence about whether to live or die.[3]

When I first read Burt, partly because of my psychoanalytic

perspective, I tended to agree with him that Dax must be ambiva-lent. But conversations with Dax, repeated viewing of *Dax's Case*, and further reflection led me to conclude that Dax may be as unam-bivalent as he claims about his own thoughts and feelings. Dax did want to die; he did want to stop treatment; he did know what he wanted. His unambiguous, unambivalent thoughts and desires were perhaps a major source of continuity between Don and Dax Cowart. He lost his body, but not his mind.

It is worth noting that Dax changed only his first name, not his entire name. This is consistent with his partial loss of personal iden-tity, and more specifically to the partial loss of his hearing. For Dax his auditory capacity is especially important because of his blind-ness. And his hearing is an essential pathway for him to relation-ships with other persons as well as to pleasure in listening to music. Dax says that should he suffer total hearing loss, he is not sure his life would be worth living any longer. Moreover, even though his body was severely damaged it was not totally destroyed. So there is a fragile physical continuity—even the continual pain reinforced the fact that his body was alive—that links Don and Dax Cowart.

Why "Dax"? I noticed that when Dax signs a document in one of the interview segments that he signs "Dax" with a flourish that emphasizes the "X." I am reminded of the remark Dr. Charles Baxter made that he had to ask Ada Cowart to sign the consent forms for treatment because Dax's hands were so severely burned that he could only make an X. But the truth is that Dax would not have consented to making an "X" or signing his name had he been physically able to do so. I don't suggest that Dax chose the name in response to Baxter. But "Dax" is a singular and intriguing choice.[4] It even retains the "D" and "a" of Donald and adds the "X." So the "X" that Dax was not permitted to make—or refused to make—on the consent forms is incorporated into his new name which he can and does sign. This symbol of independence is not insignificant.

It is curious that his mother and many others continue to speak of Don or Donnie, not Dax. In her case it may be influenced by the fact that she and her husband gave Donald his name and she feels that he has no right to discard it. She does not acknowledge the name change. Perhaps Larson used "Don" and the diminutive "Donnie" because he believed that they really did save his life and salvaged what they could of the body of Donald Cowart. But for Dax—as for Art Rousseau—Don "was dead already" and there "wasn't going to be Don Cowart anymore."

It is my view that Dax Cowart is a person who emerged with the disfigured remnants of the body of Don Cowart and the mind—scarred by the experience of pain and loss of freedom—that had been there all along. But Dax is a transformed person who has achieved a new identity. No longer capable of the physical feats of an athlete, pilot, or rodeo rider, he has gradually moved from a nearly dead victim of an explosion, to a patient in intractable pain demanding to die, to a wealthy plaintiff who settled a personal injury lawsuit against the gas company, to a depressed and dependent cripple, to a law student dropout, to a businesman, husband (now divorced), and, finally, a graduate of Texas Tech Law School and a member of the Texas Bar Association. Of course there are many more phases to Dax's development than those that I have mentioned, but they illustrate the changes in personality and transformations that help us to identify the novelty as well as the continuity in the personality of Don "Donnie" Cowart aka Dax Cowart.

FREEDOM, COMPETENCE, AND MAKING DECISIONS

A recurrent theme in *Dax's Case* concerns the many decisions that had to be made about Dax in connection with his emergency and long-term treatment and rehabilitation, his competence to choose, his desire to refuse or discontinue treatment as well as his suicidal impulses, his life-style, and his future. Although one might be tempted to describe this complex set of decisions in terms of an autonomy/paternalism framework, it is my view that the matrix of choices, values, and consequences is too complex to be characterized only by an autonomy/paternalism dichotomy. In addition, let us consider the web of relationships that linked Dax with his mother, his lawyer, and the medical staff that took care of him. I will first consider several separate relationships and then some of their interconnections.

The relationship between Dax and his mother is, of course, complex. Although my concern is with the manifestations of their relationship in the context of Dax's injury and subsequent treatment and care, we cannot ignore certain prominent features of their over-all relationship. One such feature concerns Ada Cowart's strongly held religious beliefs that provided her with support in a time of crisis and a basis for her decision to consent to the physician's request to treat Dax over his objections and against his will. Another is the natural tendency of a mother to protect her child, even from himself, especially if she believes that he lacks adequate capacity to decide for himself. She also pointed out that if treatment was stopped, such a decision would be irreversible after a certain point. She found it impossible to give up on her child—especially after she had just lost her husband. It is also clear that Ada Cowart is a woman whose tenacity in her beliefs and opinions rivals that of her son, at times locking them in a power struggle that extended well beyond treatment decisions. Included are momentous issues such as preventing Dax from attempting suicide as well as lesser questions about whether he could drink beer in her house or what clothes he should wear. From her point of view it appears that she did what she felt she had to do.

Dax, however, does not blame his mother and says that he understands her feelings. He believes that she should never have been placed in the position to make treatment decisions on his behalf, that only he should have had the right to decide. It is also possible that because Dax was certain about how she would decide, he was able to express his diametrically opposite feelings and beliefs with assurance that he would be contradicted. It may be that his relentless expression of his desire to die was the only vestige of freedom remaining to him in his captive and totally dependent condition after his injury. The power struggle with his mother was of course in part a reaction to his dependence on her, an unavoidable emotional regression in the face of his injury, and in part a reaction to his being a captive held for treatment by his physicians. I suspect that Dax knew he could rely on his mother not to abandon him no matter what he said to her.[5] He may have been less comfortable about and confident in expressing his outrage at his disability, anger at being treated, and grief over the loss of his capacities to his physicians and other medical staff—even though he did express his feelings toward them as well.

Dax perceived his relationship with Dr. Baxter to be that of a prisoner as well as a patient. Because he was so physically powerless and thought by Baxter to be incompetent, Dax was not at first taken seriously by Baxter as a person capable of making his own treatment decisions. Baxter says that he literally ignored Dax's initial request to die on the grounds that during the crisis phase of treatment Dax was in so much pain, shock, and under the influence of narcotics that his judgment could not be trusted. Later he realized how serious Dax was about wanting to die and that he was rational and competent. I suspect, however, that had Dax readily agreed to be treated, Baxter would not have questioned Dax's competence and would have allowed him to make an "X" on the consent form. It is common for physicians to question the competence of patients when the patient rejects a proposed treatment but to assume that they are competent when they consent. This is what Dr. Fritz Redlich calls the physicians' presumption that all patients are incompetent if they disagree with their doctors.

Another aspect of Baxter's view of his relationship with Dax was shaped by Baxter's idea that he had a duty to deliver medical care and Dax had a duty to receive it. Baxter, like Larson, did not have a difficult time deciding to treat because he realized that he had a chance, even though remote, to save Dax's life. It is a legitimate goal of medicine to save lives whenever possible. Baxter and Larson value that goal more highly than the right of a presumed incompetent patient to refuse treatment.[6] For that matter they believe that even if Dax was competent, he was not rational and that they had the authority to override his refusals.

From Dax's point of view, however, the value of his life was much less than the significance he ascribed to his right not to be coerced and forced to be treated and the right to make his own personal treatment choices. Dax had totally lost control of his body, his mobility, and his freedom. Given his fiercely independent spirit and pleasure in choosing his own risks—such as being a fighter pilot or a rodeo rider—the deep psychological pain of helplessness compounded the relentless and excruciating physical pain of the burns. It may well have been true that, as Baxter remarked, Dax's expression of the desire to die was aimed at getting what he wanted—the ability to control and manipulate his environment. But for Dax this meant release from the solitary confinement in his hospital prison and the torture of his physical pain. Burt notes Dax's concern about how others saw him and whether they thought he should die. Dax was also in despair because no one listened to and adequately understood what he was saying about his physical and emotional needs. I suspect that many people who encountered Dax in the early years of his treatment were ambivalent about whether they wanted him to live. What Burt interprets as Dax's ambivalence, I would see as the ambivalence of others toward him, his suffering and pain, and their doubts about his quality of life in the future. In fact, one might wonder whether the vigorous treatment of Dax masked unconscious ambivalence the staff felt toward him; they consciously used all their skills to save him while, perhaps, secretly wishing that he would die.

Dax, however, was not ambivalent—he *knew* that he wanted to die, that he believed that the quality of his future life would not make it worth living. Dax was at least making a claim about his feelings at that time about his future prospects. He probably also thought he was making an accurate, even if not an objective, prediction. Fortunately for those of us who have had the opportunity to know and learn from Dax, others—his mother and physicians—were more uncertain about his future than Dax. And though Dax's rights were violated, his expectations about a hopeless future were mistaken. This in no way negates the strong and univocal feelings Dax had at the time about his desire to die.

It was Dr. Robert White's response to Dax, in my estimation, that played a crucial role in initiating the transformation of Dax's life from helplessness, dependence, and despair to a recognition of competence and a rejuvenation of his personality—though not without long periods of depression, struggle, disappointments, and, eventually, restoration of a degree of personal freedom and accomplishment. It is important to emphasize that the declaration that Mr. Cowart, as Dr. White calls him, was a competent adult able to choose whether to receive treatment was only one aspect of their relationship. It is also essential that White understood and appreciated Dax's own feelings and point of view. For it seems that, as Art Rousseau observed, everyone wanted to keep Dax from talking, especially about his desire to die. Yet what else could Dax do to assert his identity, to be himself? White first listened, then he empathized and understood, and then determined that Dax was a competent adult. Dax was not intellectually incapacitated, not a child, not a prisoner, not an incompetent patient. Even if, to some degree, these other elements were present, from a psychological and moral perspective he was a person deserving respect. This is displayed not only in the manner in which White refers to Mr. Cowart (not Don or Donnie), but also in the manner in which White responds to him as illustrated in *Please Let Me Die*.

Dax, in turn, has since 1974 remained in periodic contact with White, come to him later for help in dealing with his sleep disturbance, and has turned to White for support and assistance—on his own terms rather than on imposed terms. Indeed when Dax was finally deemed competent he did—somewhat inexplicably—consent to the surgery proposed by Dr. Larson.[7] Whether it was—as Larson suggests—because he challenged Dax or whether it was because White recognized Dax's personal autonomy is unclear to me. It is clear, however, that the relationship between Dax and White has a quality of mutual respect rather than the paternalistic dominance of Larson and the maternal dominance of his mother.

Rex Houston also played a key role in Dax's life. Houston, as Dax's friend and attorney, advised him to pursue his lawsuit as a "live plaintiff" to collect a substantial settlement. As a family friend he also helped negotiate the later conflicts and tensions between Dax and his mother. And it appears that Houston also adopted an understandably paternalistic position toward Dax's desire to die by refusing treatment or committing suicide. Many attorneys—certainly in the mid-1970s—would have behaved like Houston, especially given his personal beliefs and his relationships with the Cowart family. Houston not only discouraged but refused to assist Dax in his quest for death. Other attorneys, especially in the mid-1980s, would adopt a position more akin to that of the attorneys for Elizabeth Bouvia (the young California woman with cerebral palsy who sought to die by starvation in a hospital), who argue vigorously for their client's preferences. But Bouvia has encountered great difficulty and resistance to efforts to carry out her death wish. Even if she, like Dax, is not ambivalent, we—and some of the judges who heard her case—inevitably are. I do not blame Houston for his unwillingness to help Dax carry out his desires even though I have difficulty in accepting his refusal to advocate Dax's position. I suspect he felt that the best he could do for Dax at the time was to help him gain financial security through the lawsuit. And in that respect he served his client well.

Dax repeatedly objects to the fact that he was forcibly treated and not respected as a competent and rational person. It appears from the interviews that most people were uncomfortable about talking or did not want to talk with Dax about his desire to die, refuse treatment, or commit suicide. His demands were dismissed as issuing from an incompetent person or were brushed aside as irrational or unacceptable. But White, at least, understood why Dax might rationally desire to die at the same time that he realized that Dax might lack adequate information about the future to be in a position to fully assess his situation. It is the importance of being understood and respected as a person capable of choosing competently—even if not necessarily rationally—that was so critical to Dax. At the close of *Dax's Case* we hear Dax say that it is the right to choose for himself and the right not to be forced to endure pain and agony that is so important to personal freedom and civil rights. I agree.

At the same time it is difficult to deny that the convictions of Dax's mother and physicians are also worthy of respect. They were unwilling to permit Dax to die because they knew the future was uncertain and they believed the pain would eventually diminish; but death is irreversible. Perhaps they could not give up on Dax because they dimly perceived—or at least hoped—Dax's restorative capacity would eventually triumph over his pain, suffering, and loss.

My view is that Dax's moral and legal rights were violated. He was competent—at least after the initial trauma—and should have been permitted to refuse treatment. Dax was mistaken, however, in his beliefs and predictions about his future quality of life. Even though Dax's mother and physicians did violate Dax's rights, they also preserved the basis of his freedom—the opportunity to make choices in the future. Thus, we can appreciate their position and their conduct while at the same time agreeing with Dax. If I were in a similar situation, I would want to choose—perhaps mistakenly or irrationally—for myself.

THE DESIRE TO DIE, REFUSING TREATMENT, SUICIDE, AND ASSISTED SUICIDE

I have already pointed out that Dax realized very soon after the accident that he was dying and already partially dead. Without aggressive medical care he surely would have died and nearly did die anyway. Given his unbelievable pain and the awareness of loss of sight and other capacities, especially his despair about whether he would ever have an intimate relationship with a woman, it is understandable to me why Dax would at that time very much want to die. There are other reasons as well—such as dependence, helplessness, despair, expected future quality of life, expense—that provide a rational basis of desiring to die quickly and painlessly. Although I am not convinced that there is, as Freud believed, a death instinct, Dax's response certainly is consistent with and provides some evidence for it. The cumulative effect of these considerations certainly pulls us in the direction acknowledging both emotional, rational, and, perhaps, biological bases for Dax's desire to die.

When the desire to die arises in the context of medical treatment, however, complexities immediately arise. Although Dax was at risk for dying, his death was not inevitable. He was critically but not irreversibly injured. His dying could not only be postponed, his injuries could be treated. If successfully treated he was a candidate for surgery and other forms of rehabilitation. The medical prognosis was grim. But prognoses are often mistaken, and, in particular, outcomes in individual cases are particularly difficult to forecast. Although some physicians are too optimistic, others are sometimes too pessimistic. Patients spread across a similar spectrum. The complex variables that interact in familiar cases of disease or injury regularly challenge our tolerance for ambiguity and our ability to accept uncertainty. If Ada Cowart and the doctors in the early stages of Dax's treatment were too aggressive and optimistic, Dax himself may have been too decisive and pessimistic. Yet the beliefs and feelings of both are understandable. Both Houston and White wisely and rightly wanted to wait and see.

When a patient expresses a strong preference to refuse treatment and a physician firmly believes the treatment is necessary to save the patient's life, it may not be possible to talk, assess, negotiate, and explore options extensively. But neither patient preferences nor physician recommendations should be followed uncritically or unreflectively. It has been my experience that many apparent crises, even life-threatening ones, permit more time for thoughtful discussion than physicians sometimes admit, though perhaps less time than philosophers might prefer. Immediate decisions may need to be made to keep options open, but in a crisis usually a series of decisions must be made and different options may be chosen at different times.[8] So it was with Dax. In the aftermath of the explosion immediate treatment was required to prevent infection. After the initial crisis was over, continued treatment was necessary. Decisions to discontinue or alter treatment were made at various points over a span of time. Over this period of time, different issues become prominent. What seemed to be lacking in Dax's treatment—though this may be an unavoidable impression because of editing of the film—was adequate discussion and assessment of options, alternative decisions, and preferences. My impression is that not only did the doctors not talk to Dax, but that he did not talk to them. They insisted on one thing and he demanded another. I saw little evidence of attempts to explain, persuade, and justify on the physicians' part and little interest in hearing them on Dax's part. If any serious effort at either understanding Dax's feelings or counseling him was made, no evidence for this appears in the film. Therefore, it is my impression that Dax's refusal of treatment was as stark as the physician's insistence upon treatment was blatant. Dominance and paternalism countered by physically powerless but verbally adversarial refusal characterized the atmosphere, hardly creating a climate of reciprocity and mutual respect.[9]

At such an impasse it is not surprising that Dax would turn to others for help. Dax was furious and frustrated with his physicians and his mother for forcing him to be treated. But to whom does one then turn for help to commit suicide? Nurse Leslie Kerr and Dax's friends felt caught in an insoluble value conflict. They recognized Dax's plight and his preference, but they were understandably unwilling to assist in his suicide. Assisted suicide, if tolerable at all, is more acceptable to us when the person requesting assistance is irreversibly terminally ill, untreatable, and of advanced age. Dax was none of these. And no one was willing—as far as I know—to assist his suicide while he was in the hospital.

Dax mentions his subsequent suicide attempts as does his mother. His dependence, helplessness, boredom, despair about a future, and frustration are easy to imagine but hard to cure. Suicide may well seem to be the only way to gain control of an apparently hopeless situation and to "achieve something, even if only peace or an end to pain."[10] For Dax the impulse to commit suicide may well have been "an attempt to transform one's existence radically."[11] The aspects of suicide related to the desire to transcend despair and hopelessness about the future and to break the bonds of powerlessness are sensitively explored in Robert Jay Lifton's *The Broken Connection*. For Dax, who had for so long been forced to endure pain inflicted on his broken and disfigured body followed by years of dependence, depression, and despair, Antonin Artaud's thoughts are relevant: "If I commit suicide, it will not be to destroy myself but to put myself back together again. Suicide will be for me only one means of violently reconquering myself, of brutally invading my being, of anticipating the unpredictable approaches of God. By suicide, I reintroduce my design in nature, I shall for the first time give things the shape of my will." [12]

From this perspective Dax's suicide attempts can be seen as efforts to bring about a transformation in his life, to restore vitality and wholeness through a decisive act of suicide. Lifton writes that

> One's ultimate involvements are so impaired that one is simply unable to imagine a psychologically livable future. Whatever future one can imagine is no better, perhaps much worse, than the present ("However low a man has sunk, he can sink even lower, and this 'can' is the object of his dread," is the way Kierkegaard put the matter. *More specifically, the suicide can create a future only by killing himself.* That is, he can reawaken psychic action and imagine vital events beyond the present only in deciding upon, and carrying through, his suicide. And for that period of time, however brief, he lives with an imagined future. [13]

Although the suicide attempts failed, the transformation did occur. As I suggested earlier, the partial name change can be seen as a response to partial death. The partial name change also symbolizes the birth of a partially new person. Years of pain and suffering, depression and despair, dependence and gradual independence, relationships with his family, friends, former wife, and others have contributed to an improvement in Dax's quality of life that he did not foresee. As the attempts at suicide reveal, the yearning for a restoration of vitality was powerful. Not quickly, but eventually this was achieved. We now know Dax as a lecturer and lawyer who will no doubt be a formidable adversary in the verbal battleground of the courts.

In this compelling drama many values and issues are at stake: the right to choose, preservation of life, quality of life, parent-child, doctor-patient, nurse-patient, and lawyer-client relationships, cognitive and emotional competence, rehabilitation, compensation for injury, the need to be listened to and understood, the unpredictability of treatment and future life choices, the limitations of physical disability and the methods of coping with them, and many others. We learn from Dax that strength of will, tenacity, and vitality can contribute to a restoration, not only of the self, but also of an acceptable quality of life. But state-of-the-art medical care, luck, money, emotional support, and understanding are also essential. Notwithstanding the violation of his rights, cure and healing can and did occur. Although the justification for their actions Dax's mother and his physicians offered are not convincing, their conduct is understandable and, though morally and legally wrong, partially excusable. Dax's piercing logic and crystal clarity when talking about the right to freedom and personal choice exemplify his intellectual vitality. His tenacity, realism, and humor reveal an emotional depth and resilience that is as inspiring as it is rare. For this reason we should admire and stand in awe of Dax's transformation and accomplishments. Most importantly, he rightly emphasizes that the competent individual's right to choose—even mistakenly—may be the most significant value we can endorse in the face of unpredictable events and uncertain outcomes in the drama of individual lives.

NOTES

1. According to Lonnie D. Kliever, Dax changed his name during the making of *Dax's Case* in 1982.

2. In a conversation with Dax on May 29, 1986, he told me that he was named after two friends of his father. Dax said that he never much cared for the name "Donald Herbert" anyway. Perhaps because his father's friends were

dead when "Dax" was born, it made sense to discard the names now that part of him was also dead.

3. Robert Burt, *Taking Care of Strangers* (New York: The Free Press, 1979), 1–22, 174–80.

4. Dax told me that he chose the name "Dax" because of the main character in Harold Robbins's *The Adventurers*, whose initials were D.A.X. In the novel, D.A.X. was, above all, a survivor of violence, physical abuse, torture, and the power of others. He survived because of tenacity, loyalty, insight, pragmatism, and a refusal to surrender his spirit. The real Dax is also a survivor, but more than that he is a man who has transcended his physical disabilities to embody a self in continuing transformation.

5. A philosopher colleague, Ray Lanfear, has written to me that the position of Dax's mother may have "enabled him to complain in what might be the most therapeutic manner. It seems to me that when human beings are stressfully pained (physically or emotionally) they mostly need to scream out against the way things are—scream out against reality, if you will. Classic tragedians captured that need, I think. (I have Euripides, Sophocles, and Shakespeare in mind.) That Dax knew he could count on his mother enabled him to express his discontent in the sharpest and most intense way. He could scream out against life itself and against the injustice of having that very life forced upon him, and he could do so sincerely, too. Yet, deep within himself he knew that his mother would not allow him to die. Perhaps that is why he is surprisingly happy now."

6. See Gary B. Weiss, "Paternalism Modernized," *Journal of Medical Ethics*, 11(1985): 184–87.

7. Robert B. White, "A Demand to Die," *Hastings Center Report* 5 (June 1975): 9–10.

8. See, generally, J. Katz, *The Silent World of Doctor and Patient* (New York: The Free Press, 1985).

9. See Ronald A. Carson, "On Rescuing and Abiding," *Texas Humanist* 6 (May–June 1984), 28.

10. Robert Jay Lifton, *The Broken Connection* (New York: Simon and Schuster, 1983), 256.

11. Ibid., 252.

12. Ibid.

13. Ibid., 249–50.

Dealing with Catastrophe 🜍
William F. May

THE EDITOR OF THIS BOOK ON *DAX'S CASE* SENT
me the film some five months before I could bring myself to watch
it. The reason for delay goes deeper than the busy teacher's tendency
to procrastinate on writing assignments. My past record on burn
cases suggests a more troubling reserve than an aversion to work.
Some ten years ago, while spending a sabbatical year as an observer
on various hospital services, I made arrangements to visit the burn
unit, but somehow I managed not to get there. My lack of courage,
then and now, blurts out a major problem that Dax and all who
have suffered catastrophic burns face daily—long after the surgeons
have done their best and produced what they consider a technical
success. The scarred patient must cope with the aversion of others.

This aversive behavior shows up variously. Strangers stare
rudely or quickly avert their eyes as they recognize the magnitude of
what they have seen. Professionals at work in the crisis centers—
nurses, social workers, and other therapists—burn out after six
months or so. Acquaintances and colleagues manage to stabilize
their behavior through regular contact, but the plight of the victim
still sends a deep tremor through their lives. Meanwhile, family
members and friends obsess themselves with an event that has irrevocably altered a portion of their lives.

But the deepest aversion besets the victims. They know that their very existence produces an aversive recoil in others, which long precedes any and all discrete interactions. Moreover, helplessness in the midst of these uncontrollable impacts produces a second generation of responses somewhat less innocent than the first. The foolish inspire contempt; the nervous, impatience; the transient philanthropists and tourists, anger; and friends and professionals, the temptation to manipulate. No sensitive patients can fail to note their own unsavory responses and more. Thus they experience a profound aversion not only to the event but also to themselves. Neither the technical successes of medicine nor the company of others can touch the problem. For in leaving them disfigured, medicine leaves them with a chronic sorrow, a limitless grief, which the aversive swoons of others salute but cannot heal.

Dax himself goes to the heart of the event in an interview some eleven years after the explosion and fire that took his father's life and severely burned two-thirds of his own body, including his face, his eyes, his ears, and his hands, leaving charred flesh and scorched earth where, an instant before, functioned a twenty-five-year-old man. This young man, recently discharged from the service where he served as a jet pilot, had already excelled as a golfer, surfer, football player, trackman, and rodeo performer. Like so many other burn victims, he remained wholly conscious during the disaster. He thought, while cutting through three walls of fire, rolling on the ground, and running again, "It couldn't be happening—a dream, a nightmare—but it really was happening." The first man on the scene, a farmer, exclaimed, "O my God" and Dax said, "Go help my father" and then asked the farmer for a gun. "Don't you see, I am a dead man. I can't live."

That horrific assessment goes to the heart of Dax's problem. He does not say "I am dying." Such a prediction would have to yield in due course to the superior knowledge of the medical experts who would lift his untouchable body by his belt, take him to the hospital, and eventually conclude there, "No, we can keep you alive." Dax says, rather, "I am (already) a dead man." Whatever that dreadful pronouncement means, it insists that human life is not mere biological life. (Dax, after all, is sufficiently alive at that moment to judge himself dead.) And human death is not, pure and simple, its biological termination.

But, at the same time, Dax's self-appraisal exposes the shallowness of all those efforts to interpret catastrophe by appeal to the category of quality of life. Don Cowart knows that he has not simply suffered a modification in his quality of life, some changes at the margins of his life; the explosion has annihilated him. Don Cowart, as defined by everything that he was, has died.

This experience of burn as death, moreover, includes not only the original catastrophe but also its inevitable biological consequences, the ordeal of medical treatment, and the end results of that treatment. Death turns out to be not a single episode but an enforced and reinforced condition. We will need, therefore, to look not simply at Dax's condition when he pronounces himself dead but at the full outworking of that event. This essay will attempt to interpret this state of affairs and its implication for all those who face, or care for those facing, catastrophe.

INSTANT IMPAIRMENT OF FUNCTION

Dax loses on the instant one eye completely, two-thirds of his skin, including his eyelids, his face, his ears, the skin on his hands and legs. Unlike other burn victims, he does not appear to have suffered from smoke inhalation which would compromise his breathing. He does not suffer brain damage or the loss of consciousness (though in the ensuing treatment, he will experience what the literature refers to as psychotic breaks, as he hallucinates and imagines the worst of the nursing staff). We can assume that he can still smell and taste (though what he smells of burned tissue and, ultimately, of infection will offend himself and others). He cannot walk, he cannot use his hands, and he cannot touch or be touched.

These various losses, quite apart from the complexities and rigors of treatment to come, will blast that identity which each of us assumes with our bodies as the instrument of mastery. The explosion and fire destroy Dax the fighter pilot and Dax the athlete. They also annihilate, at least temporarily, the sluice gate of the senses. Nurse Leslie E. Einfeldt of the University of Washington Burn Center reports more generally about the severely burned patient, "All five of his senses have not only been overwhelmingly assaulted but have been rendered temporarily inoperative."[1] This fearsome assault continues in the intensive care unit of the burn center,

> where every available orifice and some newly created apertures . . . [are] cannullated. He . . . [is] connected to a vast array of machines each with its own lights, sounds, and motions, all of which are totally foreign to the patient. Every breath is tainted with the smell of burnt tissue and reminds him of the accident. He cannot see, hear, nor taste in a normal manner. He cannot touch nor sense touch due to his damaged receptors. With the complexity and intensity of care he will require, his sleep pattern will undoubtedly be altered.[2]

Einfeldt's description emphasizes the way in which the original blast continues, as it were, even in the effort to treat and heal. Healing continues to assault the senses and impair function. (The third-degree patient temporarily loses the sense of pain through the body surface, but the healing of tissue reactivates, with a vengeance, the capacity to experience pain, and it can also, through the contracture of scar tissue, further constrict movement and function.) The patient senses not simply death, but that the staff continues, as it were, the killing process.

THE ASSAULT OF TREATMENT

The emergency room staff needs to establish immediately an airway for breathing, restore circulatory volume to prevent shock, and, if possible, to evaluate promptly the patient's mental status, since, as Nurse Gay G. Hayward has noted,[3] the patient will likely communicate less readily soon thereafter. Initially the patient may suffer no airway obstruction; he or she may be able to speak, especially if he or she is not hypoxic or has not suffered an inhalation injury that harms the air saccules in the lungs. However, during the six to twelve hours after arrival in the burn unit, patients often experience laryngeal edema; the head and neck swell to grotesque, pumpkin-like proportions; eschar leave the surface appearing like a puffed up, decomposing body. The emergency room staff will intubate the patients to prevent certain death, robbing them, while conscious, of their main means of communicating with the world. The tube remains in place for three or more days until the edema subsides. In the interim, the patient is likely to hear a staff member say, "I'm going to roll you, okay?" or "I have to change your folly, okay?" The patient lies there in the midst of these well-meaning efforts to elicit consent with a French plastic tube down the throat and with all vital functions on the assist control of the ventilator.

The staff also installs intravenous lines to provide nourishment and to cope with a major crisis in the functioning of the circulatory system. The standard 154-pound man requires a daily fluid maintenance of three liters to compensate for the fluid losses through urine, sweat, and breathing. Ordinarily, the body enjoys a delicate homeostasis, a splendid harmony, which the skin serves by clothing the body. The skin functions as the boundary between the self and its world. It keeps the precious within and the noxious without. It prevents fragile protoplasm from oozing into the surroundings and serves as a barrier to invading microorganisms. It regulates temperature and fluid loss and keeps deeper body functions in balance. Pimply in youth, wrinkled in age, the skin defines our extended selves, our health, and our limits.

The person with full thickness burns over 50 percent of the body suffers a rude shock to this integral functioning. The durable elastic barrier which holds precious fluids within, through which he or she experiences the pleasures of the universe, and which keeps destruction and decomposition at bay, burns away, annihilating cell membranes. Unable to prevent evaporation, the body loses massive amounts of fluids. The *minimum* fluid requirements may leap from three liters to fourteen liters in the first twenty-four hours following a 50 percent, third-degree burn. The body reacts by descending into the deep physiological shock of hypovolemia. Cell walls destroyed, the body starts to ooze its precious plasma. Somehow the body must cope with this depletion just as the burn accelerates the victim's metabolic rate, further increasing the need for food.

Regrettably, the initial widespread breach of the body's surface extends itself inward, forcing successive waves of collapse compromising further walls, protective mechanisms, and body functions. The hypovolemic shock produces tiny ulcerations in the gastrointestinal tract with some sloughing of the gastric mucosa. A paralysis ensues in the intestinal tract, making it impossible for the patient to process food. Not only does the world about recoil, but the digestive system profoundly recoils and comes to a halt. The patient may also experience a kind of psychological equivalent of this intestinal recoil with the onset of depression and anorexia.

These factors singly and in combination necessitate intravenous feeding, which dumps massive amounts of fluid into the leaking tank of the body in an effort to nourish and protect other organs. This strategy, however, endangers in other ways the quality of the patient's recovery. Intravenous fluids increase the swelling at already bloated points of entry and overload the kidneys which have suffered a reduction in their capacity to process fluid. The general swelling, in turn, blocks circulation, hampers healing, and threatens the patient with the destruction of more skin. The staff, in brief, works with contrary pressures upon it in the midst of crisis, and the patient suffers treatments which, while necessary to save life, severely limit one another.

TUBBING, PAIN, AND COLD

The staff fights the bacterial invasion, to which the destruction of the body's borders and the weakening of its immunological capacities expose the patient, by cleansing wounds, cutting away dead or contaminated tissue (debridement), removing scales, handling other nonviable tissues by enzymatic removal, and repeatedly applying salves to the wounds, and changing dressings. In addition to these painful procedures, the staff subjects the patient to daily tubbings. Immersion aids in preventing infection and in removing water-soluble, cream-based dressings, dead skin, and crusts. Daily tubbing also facilitates joint motion and thus helps preserve those functions necessary to mastery and control. The staff during tubbing keeps the room temperature at 80 degrees Fahrenheit and the water temperature at 98.5 to 100 degrees. The patient complains of shivering. Robbed of its natural clothing, the body suffers a severe reduction in its ability to regulate its own temperature. Meanwhile, staff members work at room temperatures much too hot for their own comfort. They find themselves inflicting cold while they themselves are insufferably warm.

At the same time, tubbing causes pain so excruciating that one surgeon advises hospital architects to remove the tank room far from the burn unit beds so as to reserve the patient's bed as a respite from the place of torture and, in a phrase that speaks volumes, to avoid "sensitizing the other patients."[4]

Not that the burn victim escapes pain away from the tubbing room. Partial thickness burns release prostaglandins and histamines around the injured area that cause pain. Exposure to the air causes pain. Heterotopic bone forming in the joints causes deep pain, and the stretching of contractures also causes pain. Burn victims continue to experience pain even after their wounds heal; in this respect, they resemble the arthritic patient who remains sensitive to changes in the weather. All strategies to manage pain also have their limits, whether by hypnosis, acupuncture, or drugs. While the pain caused by partial thickness burns will respond to nonopiate prostaglandin inhibitors, the pain resulting from full thickness burns in the course of tubbing treatment responds only partly to opiate analgesics.

Perhaps more than any other feature of illness, pain helps render patients anomic; it disconnects them from the ordinary patterns and rhythms of life. Those patterns are shot through with meaning and purpose, partly immediate and partly ultimate. Pain disconnects. The body, which we largely take for granted in the pursuit of ends, suddenly obtrudes and distracts from our goals, as it recoils protectively from, or writhes in the midst of, pain. The toothache, the throbbing headache, nausea, the scorched body— these pains take over; they isolate us from community and they disorient us from the arena of ends. Pain, in the jargon of one author, is "telic dysfunctional." It effects the decentralization of the "higher telos of the organism, and its loss of dominance over the lower tele,"[5] a state which Jesus expressed more bluntly, "My God, my God, why hast thou forsaken me?"

POSITIONING AND SPLINTING

The eventual acquisition of scar tissue reclothes the body but with a material too thick and contracting to permit normal movement at the joints. As a wound heals, the tissue pulls tight until it meets an opposing force; patients find a contracted position most comfortable. Unless opposed, scars over the joints of the shoulder, elbow, hands, hips, knees, or feet massively shrink, immobilize, and deform. Scars present children with even greater problems since the fixed, thick surface does not accommodate for the growing body (particularly acute for the young girl with a scarred chest whose breasts begin to bud). A deep burn on the front of the neck (whether afflicting an adult or child), will pull down the patient's chin to the chest, affecting not only looks but ability to eat without drooling. To counteract the chin's descent into the chest, the staff will position the patient's head back over the edge of a mattress. Dorsal burns on the hands quickly contract, creating the so-called burned claw hand, at once severely crippling and deforming.[6] Palmar burns similarly render the hand useless. A regimen of positioning, splinting, and frequent exercise may reduce the need for still further reconstructive surgery at a later date on crucial joints. To be sure, the medical staff can do a great deal to restore or to find surrogates for function. Dax can now type—albeit with his tongue, not with fingers. But the severely burned patient, under the best of circumstances, suffers a permanent alteration in ability to master, control, and enjoy the world. It assaults the core sense of self.

"Now, at best, I couldn't do the things I really enjoy. I'd have to change completely the things that I'm interested in. It isn't likely that I'd become interested in things I wasn't interested in before."[7]

DISFIGUREMENT

The surgeons concede that, while they can restore some function, they can do much less to restore appearance. The language of the experts sometimes retreats here into the euphemistic. Dr. John D. Constable's sensitive essay on disfigurement hides under the stilted title "Limitations of Aesthetic Reconstruction." The editors of the volume *Comprehensive Approaches to the Burned Person* discreetly tuck away this chapter at the end of the book. But the starkness of the limitations upon the healing arts breaks out in sentence after sentence in this and other essays: "The ultimate or final reconstruction of the severely burned face can be expected to remain, if not positively repellent and grotesque, at least unsatisfactory and unpleasing."[8] Or again, "The surgeon must accept that what delights him as a technical result may still be a horror to his patient."[9] And most poignantly, "Our work requires putting a new facial garment, often a garment of sorrow, on these patients."[10]

Constable chooses his metaphor carefully. Rehabilitation in its Latin root, *habil*, means to clothe. The soul, in a sense, never exposes itself utterly naked. It presents itself to another in and through the body, the soul's clothing, as it were, the medium of its veiling, unveiling. In their first stages of hope, family members bring to the surgeon earlier pictures of the burned victim to assist in the restoration. But, whatever rehabilitation means, it cannot restore. Not that the surgeon's art lacks ingenuity. (He or she may cover the patient temporarily with allograft and xenograft skin or amniotic membranes or the synthetic covering Biobrane and, of course, autogenous skin, where available.)[11] But, even at best, making full use of pressure garments to flatten the thick surface and to soften scar lines, the surgeon cannot, in the case of severe facial burns, restore looks. That term, of course, still misses the point. The patient's "look" is not an abstract object of aesthetic judgment. It is always *someone's* look and therefore cuts to the core of *self*-presentation. An alien has now taken over that presentation. A casement has replaced the soul's own clothing. Hence, the burned child sometimes is teased and called a "mummy."

Victims feel wholly vulnerable and therefore ashamed. The visual impact on others flies out ahead, beyond control. They cannot count on the serendipity of interaction with others. Their disfigurement stiffens in advance their response. Thus the scar not only encases and distorts the victim; in a sense, it also encases and distorts the responses of others, a predicament which they solve by avoidance. Physical therapist Nancy Hansen reports of a group of adolescent burn patients that the problem of reentering society preoccupied them more than any other consequence of their accident. Dax comments eleven years after his injuries, "Because of my disfigurement, I wondered whether I would ever have a meaningful relationship with the opposite sex. I considered not going out in public at all. Finally, I had such a bad case of cabin fever, I said, to hell with it. Though it was easier for me because I couldn't see. It would be harder for somebody who wasn't blind." [12]

LIFE VS. QUALITY OF LIFE

At first glance, Dax's case seems to fit the conventional patterns of controversy in medical ethics. Most of the moral issues in medicine today turn on the conflicts between two rival values—life vs. quality of life—and between two rival principles for determining the relevant decision maker—paternalism vs. autonomy. Pro-lifers hold to life as the supreme good and oppose any and all decisions to terminate life on the basis of changes in the quality of one's life. Dax, on the other hand, appears to join those who invoke the principle of quality of life when pleading with his mother and his managers to allow him to die.

This substantive dispute between the values of life and quality of life quickly shifts into a procedural controversy over the identity of the relevant decision maker. Dax's doctors and the medical establishment as a whole tend to fight unconditionally for life.

Therefore, Dax must contest their legitimacy as decision makers. He invokes the principle of autonomy, to assert his right of self-determination, and inveighs against the preemptive and paternalistic action of the medical staff.

Dax's case, however, challenges this conventional anlaysis of the great moral issues in medical ethics. When we see the basic issue in medical catastrophe as a conflict between the values of life and quality of life, we make a series of false assumptions. First, we think of life in unilinear terms. We imagine it a straight line that begins with birth and that concludes with biological death. The line has a beginning and an end. All else in between we characterize by the substantive: life. Not that the line itself is changeless. Living creatures undergo, through their own making and through fate and fortune, a series of modifications for which we reserve the term quality of life. Sometimes, the line fattens and we think of the subject's quality of life as good; at other times, it thins out and we will characterize the quality of life as poor. A varying quality of life simply suggests variations in the same substantive—life. It allows for qualifications or modifications, but no more—until life comes to its end.

The current formulation of the debate between pro-lifers and pro-quality-of-lifers obscures the plight of Dax and others who have suffered a major illness or trauma. Traumatized persons do not experience their lives as a continuous straight line that will eventually terminate in biological death. The catastrophic event or series of events has already confronted them as annihilating. The lifeline has already broken, whether through a single event, a series of events, or a single event that unfurls a series of secondary and devastating consequences in its wake including the ordeal of treatment. The highway accident, the devastating fire, the mental breakdown of a family member, the irreversible, progressive, and immobilizing disease transform the substance of one's existence; they do not merely qualify life at its edges. The category of quality of life, with its notion of variations, positive and negative, on a rather continuous scale, simply fails to reflect actual experience. One deals not with a continuous line that thickens and thins, depending upon circumstances, but with the experience of definitive, substantive break.

The patient faces, then, an existential problem that the conventionally posed quandary of life vs. quality of life does not touch: how does one respond to one's death, to a total, comprehensive, all-penetrating, sun-blackening, oxygen-removing, flesh-charring, chilling, stilling, benumbing, and isolating death? If there is any life after such events, it will depend upon radical reconstruction from the ground up, upon the accession to new power, and the appropriation of patterns that define a new existence. One cannot talk simply of a new accessory here, a change of venue there, but of a new Phoenix that must emerge from the ashes.

A conceptual difficulty emerges. Does it make sense to use the term "dead" for the state we are describing? When Dax says, "I am a dead man," does not an "I" still exist that pronounces the verdict? Is not the word "death" used metaphorically and melodramatically, rather than realistically, to describe his state and condition? How can one talk about destruction of a substance when the substance still persists under the name Dax? Does not common sense tell us to relegate any and all changes experienced along the way to qualifications of life, no more?

The conceptual difficulty recedes if we recognize that human existence is ecstatic in the sense that the biological line alone does not define it. Individuals largely derive their existence from that which lies beyond. They try to secure their existence, to be sure, in and through the capacities, powers, and assets within their disposition and control, but, in fact, the living of life pitches them out beyond themselves into the world they savor, the several communities to which they attach themselves, and above all else, to those patterns and powers that bestow upon them meaning and that establish the rhythm, tempo, and round to their daily lives. Strip them of any and all of these and they suffer a fundamental break in existence that besets them with death.

Correspondingly, any therapist who merely tinkers with the

details of things—we can get you a typewriter that you can work with your teeth or braces that will help you stand up; or we can do another series of operations that will retrieve some thumb-finger opposition in your hand, or we can simulate some eyebrows for you— all these technical accomplishments, proffered by the surgeon and varied therapists, may significantly improve quality of life, but their triviality will only embitter patients if they themselves have not shifted over from an old identity beyond recovery to new selves on the other side of the ashes. Their problem is radical reconstruction from the ground up and not merely patchwork that attempts to obscure or minimize the loss. Only then can they take and accept and find any cause for celebration in this or that trinket that medical ingenuity can offer.

DEATH, TRANSITION, AND REBIRTH

Is there any precedent for this very different interpretation of the patient's problem that breaks with the linearism of Western medicine and Western society as a whole? In my judgment, a much older tradition of healing, based on a very different sense of human existence, supplies the more adequate alternative. Traditional societies, if we follow Arnold van Gennep and Gerhard van der Leeuw,[13] did not view life as a straight line, bounded on one side by birth and on the far side by death. Rather, death (and birth) intersected the line throughout. Periodically, men and women in traditional societies experienced the coming to an end of life as it was. They had to doff, as it were, the identity which was theirs, suffer a perilous period of transition, unclothed, until they entered into a new estate, defined by a new identity, a new pattern of life, and accession to new power. "Birth, naming, initiation, marriage, sickness and recovery, the start and end of a long journey, the outbreak of war and conclusion of peace, death and burial are all points of contact between Power and life."[14] One interprets them inadequately as mere events. They require celebration, but not in our trivializing, modern sense of that term. They entail rites of detachment from the past, rites of transition across a period of acute vulnerability, and rites of incorporation into a new estate. Not only traditional societies but also Christianity use the language of death/resurrection to emphasize the sharpness of the break between the old and the new. The metaphor of undressing and dressing expresses both ceremonially and substantively the alterations demanded of the self.

Similarly, the human ordeal we have been trying to describe in the course of this essay entails most exactingly the destruction of the soul's clothing, the imposition of a period in which the self is unclothed, and then, God willing, the painful acquisition of a new self. The surgeon may be competent to graft skin, but his or her skill alone will not avail to reclothe the soul.

The interpretation herein offered of burn patients applies more broadly to the victims of all sorts of catastrophes. The victim of a major heart attack, the couple that gives birth to a retarded child, the biopsy that announces an invasive tumor—all these events produce an upheaval, with or without rites, that disrupts daily rhythms, dashes hopes, and revises one's sense of oneself and one's past.

Shifting the key terms of the discussion from life vs. quality of life to life/death/rebirth influences a number of other issues in health care and health care ethics:

(1) It affects the resolution of the traditional quandary as to whether one should allow the patient to die. The conventional formulation of the debate—life vs. quality of life—tilts the argument in favor of the pro-lifers. The term "quality of life" does not sufficiently appreciate the destructive impact of an accident on the core self. Even a major accident seems to affect only the circumstances of life, the accidents of the self, as it were, rather than its substance. The language predisposes one powerfully in favor of continuing life under any and all circumstances. This predisposition has, in fact, ruled the medical profession. The profession has tended to define itself by an unconditional fight against biological death, without appreciating the full magnitude of the continuing death that it has imposed on the patient. In the worst of burn cases, the patient has faced two catastrophes: the first, the original burn; the second, the

catastrophe of medical survival, a catastrophe which the term "diminished quality of life" does not begin to comprehend.

(2) The very distinction between life and quality of life not only tilts the resolution of the quandary in favor of life, it also tends to slight the provision of follow-up resources to support the patient, inasmuch as that support affects only questions of life's quality. We have developed, of course, follow-up modes of care for patient rehabilitation, but the spread sheets on our allocation of resources clearly indicate that the health care dollar goes largely for acute care and only minimally for rehabilitative and chronic care.

Neglecting to provide adequate follow-up resources may in the long run weaken the support for the original decision in favor of life.

Support for the quality of one's life at first does not compete with the claim of biological life itself. Thus the community feels free to relegate questions of life's quality to the individual's own resource and responsibility. The community feels it has done its job once it has behaved like vigilantes in the protection of biological life per se. This callousness eventually produces, however, a moral and political revulsion against the pro-life movement. The language of life/death/rebirth, to the contrary, makes it clear that the responsibility of the community has just begun if it has imposed continuance upon the individual in the midst of what the individual can only experience as a living death.

(3) Concretely, the language of rebirth and reconstruction requires the community to invest much more heavily in rehabilitative and chronic care. It would also enlarge the relevant interventionists from purely medical staff to other healers, including nurses, social workers, physical therapists, occupational therapists, chaplains, and other patients who have survived similar ordeals. The technical interventions of the surgeon and the physician do not begin to touch the problems that the patient and the patient's family face. Technique supplies means to ends; but the patient faces a crisis in the ends themselves. Other health care practitioners, pastors, family

members, and the patients who have crossed the same terrain may help the patient more than practitioners of merely technical skill. These less glamorous figures may loom larger to the degree that language highlights the task of reconstruction and rebirth.

(4) This emphasis on the language of reconstruction and rebirth also forces one to recognize that the chief figure in the cast of characters is neither the surgeon nor other health care practitioners but patients themselves. Further, the old notions of ethics as a matter of problem solving fails to reckon fully with the task the patient faces. The doctor, the plumber, and the expert may puzzle over problems to solve. Once solved, they move on to other puzzles. In the process they may acquire more experience and therefore expertise, but they themselves do not substantially change. In a sense, they have no history; no self-transformation is at issue.

Patients, however, who move from life to death and some sort of new identity and rebirth make history thereby. They shape their own narrative. In the course of that shaping, they will, to be sure, need to cope with problems. But those problems are not the real issue. They themselves pose the problem. A doctor solves problems, but those problems, except at the technical level, make no further personal demands. Solving a problem provides the physician with a release from tension. Once solved, he or she no longer "agonizes" over it. Ethics in this setting is unheroic—not in that it includes no element of agony, but in that agonizing is a temporary phase of decision making from which, in a given case, one expects release. But, not so for the patient. When the staff has long since done its work and snatched the patient from the jaws of biological death, the agony, the suffering, of the patient has just begun. Thrown out into a no-man's-land, without much resource from his or her former life, cut off from former goals, old skills suddenly irrelevant, aspirations utterly unattainable, old identities and enthusiasms on the ash heap, the old persona unwearable, and the familiar rhythms and tempo of life faltering, such an individual faces vastly more than a quandary to be solved. In an unheroic age, the survivor must unexpectedly push out into the unknown, where each day is an agony, without a new identity in place.

(5) An emphasis on the language of reconstruction and rebirth does not eliminate the traditional problem of paternalism in medicine, that is, the tendency of the medical staff to limit the knowledge and the freedom of the patient for the patient's own good.

Indeed, one might argue that it intensifies the problem. If a patient merely suffers a change in the quality of his or her life, then one assumes substantial continuity between two estates. But, if one talks about an alteration in substance, then one might begin to argue that the patient is in no position to make judgments about a possible new identity and estate. A decision maker is needed, acting for him or her in the absence of a newly established center of being. Thus Dax's case and many lesser catastrophes continue to raise the question of paternalism vs. autonomy, whether one resorts to the language life vs. quality of life or death and rebirth.

Dax, of course, did not want to move out into that no-man's-land. He said to his handlers, "Please let me die." When they refused to let him die, he accused them of paternalistic behavior. Paternalism consists of any interference, manipulation, or bypassing of the freedom of another adult which one justifies on the ground that this intrusion will best serve the patient's welfare.

No criticism of paternalistic behavior ought to dismiss altogether the value of the paternal (or parental) image that lies behind paternalism. The parental metaphor validly highlights the importance of self-sacrifice, compassion, and a kind of providential care that good diagnosis, prognosis, and therapy require in health care.

But paternalism goes beyond highlighting those important virtues in the care giver and asserts the practitioner's total sovereignty over the patient. For the sake of well-being, paternalists override the patient's freedom; they do too much; they commit the sins of the overbearing. (Correspondingly, antipaternalists can lapse into the opposing vices of the underbearing. In reducing professionals to technicians, they may do too little. They replace the paternalist's sins of commission with the minimalist's sins of omission. The practitioner offers merely technical services without the important personal ingredients of truly effective care.) At one level, of course, Dax's paternalistic managers fall into some of the selfsame sins of omission. While they insisted on continuing treatment, they identified that treatment with largely technical services which only perpetuated the horror without dealing with Dax's real problem, the problem that he had died and that neither he nor the purveyor of technical services could begin to reconstruct his life.

The chief fault of the paternalistic position is illustrated with a vengeance in A. Napier Baker's article on comprehensive approaches to the burned person.[15] The author meticulously interprets the work of the burn team in familial and paternalistic terms. The total staff, Baker asserts, constitutes the "burn center family." The burn center director assumes the role of the patriarch; the head nurse, that of the matriarch; the nurse in charge, the elder sister; assorted other members of staff serve as siblings, aunts, uncles, and cousins. Mr. Baker reserves to the patient the role of the newly arrived baby. "The burned person enters into the family having experienced severe trauma. The major insult to his system and person leaves him in a state of forced dependency. He is introduced to his new family through the painfully cleansing experience of the Hubbard tank. It is as though the first changing of his diaper were marked by repeated pin sticks."[16] Members of the burned person's biological family, the author likens to fiancees, that is, to outsiders, whom the family tests in various ways before granting membership. Baker does not invoke the parental analogy merely to emphasize the dreadful physical dependency that the disaster imposes. He then tracks after the patient through the various stages of growth—the defiant toddler, the demands and bargaining associated with toilet training, the childish demand for attention at bedtime ("Why don't they ever burn their bell fingers?" one staff member moans who serves as the author's illustration of negative parenting), and the turbulences of adolescence. Finally, the patient graduates from the burn unit, that is, "goes off to college."

The essay hardly deserves attention, except that it exposes with pedantic thoroughness the impossibility of the parental metaphor as final arbiter of the relation between the health care team and those patients who have suffered major loss. Parents have acquired their authority because they have already experienced in their own time what the infant/child/adolescent goes through. They have already endured what must come to all, one way or another, in the course of their maturation. By this standard, older, more experienced members of the health care team may reasonably adopt a benignly paternalistic attitude toward new, inexperienced members of the health care team itself, but *not* toward the burn victim. The accident, originally, and the awesome treatment, subsequently, have nothing to do with an ordinary process of maturation, least of all with a maturation that team members themselves have experienced. Rather the double catastrophe pushes out the patient into the terrain of the extraordinary—into an experience of extraordinary deprivation, intense and mercilessly regimented pain, and social hurdles that would send most caretakers themselves into stunned retreat. The domestic analogy is all wrong.

The patient, for better or worse, resembles not the balky toddler, in the bosom of the family, but rather the hero in Greek tragedy, a term which I apply not in order to flatter the patient, but simply in order to locate him. He or she bears the mark of the uncanny, the German term for which is the "*Unheimlich*," the one not at home, the one driven out beyond the ordinary precincts of hearth and city gates, where no man or woman would want to venture, and who therefore sends a tremor through the rest of the community.

Don Cowart becomes Dax Cowart. One may criticize such a person, but one cannot rightly patronize him. Should he choose to live, he is not choosing his old life. He must become another man. No parentalist can force him down that road. No mere medical technician ever does enough to assist him along that road. It requires an interior transformation, it requires ethics at the deepest level, not trivial problem solving, but the reordering of one's identity from the ground up. Nothing less than that is required of the patient who moves from saying "Please let me die" to "I am glad to be alive." That heroic movement does not vindicate his doctors, because the deeper decision was his, and only as it is his do we see in him more than a patient encased and obscured by the surgeon's art but the uncanny radiance of a man.

NOTES

1. Norman R. Bernstein, M.D., and Martin C. Robson, M.D., eds., *Comprehensive Approaches to the Burned Person*, Leslie E. Einfeldt, "Comprehensive Nursing" (New Hyde Park, N.Y.: Medical Examination Publishing Co., Inc., 1983), 118.

2. Ibid.

3. Ibid., Gay G. Hayward, "The Challenge of Burn Nursing," 78–88.

4. Ibid., Martin C. Robson, M.D., "Reconstruction and Rehabilitation from Admission: A Surgeon's Role at Each Phase," 42.

5. David Bakan, *Disease, Pain, and Sacrifice* (Boston: Beacon Press, 1971), 32.

6. Bernstein and Robson, eds., *Comprehensive Approaches*, Nancy Newton Hanson, RPT, "Practice and Planning in Physical Therapy," 177.

7. *Please Let Me Die*, Department of Educational Television, University of Texas Medical Branch, Galveston, 1974.

8. Bernstein and Robson, eds., *Comprehensive Approaches*, John D. Constable, M.D., "The Limitations of Aesthetic Reconstruction," 285.

9. Ibid., 288.

10. Ibid., 285.

11. Ibid., Robson, "Reconstruction and Rehabilitation," 43.

12. *Dax's Case*, Concern for Dying, Inc., New York, 1985.

13. Arnold van Gennep, *Rites of Passage* (Chicago: University of Chicago Press, 1972); Gerhard van der Leeuw, *Religion in Essence and Manifestation*, I, chapter 22, "Sacred Life" (New York: Harper Torch Book, 1963).

14. Ibid., 192–93.

15. Bernstein and Robson, eds., *Comprehensive Approaches*, A. Napier Baker, "Pastoral Care," 259.

16. Ibid.

Remembered in the Body: Pain and Moral Uncertainty
Sally Gadow

I

THE STORY OF DAX COWART REMAINS A DISTURB-
ing one long after reaching an outcome that many would judge satisfactory. Why has this individual's struggle the power to move us
even when, by conventional standards, it has attained a happy ending? Why should his experience involve a degree of moral anguish
so profound as to persist, years afterward, unassuaged?

Those who followed Dax's situation from the beginning expected moral uncertainty eventually to subside. Ethics classes discussing the case invariably demanded to know how it "turned out,"
with the confidence with which we open today's newspaper to learn
whether yesterday's guess for 5-across was correct. Baffling as the
case seemed initially, it was assumed that the years would prove one
side or the other right, that a decade into the story, one side would
have silenced the other. Either rehabilitation would fail and Dax be
proved right: he should have been allowed to die. Or his life would
succeed in terms of independence, friendships, career; his oppo-
nents then would be vindicated and Dax silenced.

But a decade of watching the outcome emerge has not seen either side proven right. This is not because the outcome could not be

predicted and thus might have been different (and could yet be different in another ten years). It is because, although the results happen to be in his favor, Dax remains unreconciled to the means used to attain them. Even if his present well-being could have been foreseen with certainty, he nonetheless would regard his treatment as wrong. The memory of the means becomes part of its outcome. "What is remembered in the body is well remembered, and that no consent was given in this massive sentient alteration is likely to be part of what is remembered. Thus it is possible that rather than an acceptance of outcome there would instead be an indifference . . . a rebellion."[1]

The moral disagreement between Dax and proponents of his treatment has not abated. By now it appears that neither arbitration nor a different outcome would bring agreement. The intrinsic moral ambiguity of causing pain without permission has not been dissolved, and it is that ambiguity that keeps the anguish of Dax's case from subsiding finally into the silence of moral certainty. The most elegant ethical reasoning cannot erase the ambiguity, because no argument on behalf of Dax's good can fail to address the reality that, in addition to good—or instead of it—serious harm was done.

The harm consisted of the suffering forced upon him by those who insisted upon treatment. No one able to recognize the crushing power of Dax's pain would belittle it, would argue that physical harm was not caused (that, on the contrary, the painful tubbings cleansed and not damaged the tissue), that neither was moral harm inflicted, because the pain served the interest of an otherwise unattainable value. The premise that pain is a real, objective harm is a fundamental axiom of medicine, so the obscenity of denying its significance in Dax's case would be surprising, despite the fact that in academic arguments about the case it is not uncommon to hear the pain diminished, the ambiguity erased. As much as Dax and those around him may have longed to remove the ambiguity, it would have been impossible to do so by ignoring the pain.

As soon as pain is acknowledged to be a serious harm, only the most extreme moral interpretations can resolve the ambiguity of medicine as its agent. In the following discussion I will examine two of those interpretations. Although I will use the designations "Dax" and "his therapists" to refer to participants in any situation like this one, no inference is implied that individuals in Dax's own case held either of those views. To the extent that Dax and those around him tried to make sense of his pain by removing its moral ambiguity, the two views I describe were available to them but were not necessarily adopted.

The moral views to which participants can be driven in a case such as this one will seem fanatic and implausible until the situation itself is understood. Before turning in sections III and IV to moral interpretations of Dax's pain, it is important first to portray the existential complexities in the relationship between Dax and his therapists. When those have been elaborated, it will be evident how radically disparate are the experiences of the two sides and how single-minded, if not fanatic, the attempts may be to make moral sense of the situation that forces them together.

II

> Whatever their spatial proximity there are no two experiences farther apart than suffering and inflicting pain. . . . Person and person confront one another across the intermediate fact that one is embodied and the other disembodied, an intermediate fact that makes mediation for a time impossible.[2]

The distance between Dax and his therapists can be summarized as the difference between, in his case, having the body as one's entire—and entirely negative—sphere of existence and, in their case, freely functioning without regard for the possible torments of embodiment. Each of these states is a distortion of the two realms between which experience normally moves: alternately becoming so absorbed by activities that the body is forgotten, then being recalled to it by hunger, fatigue, or other physical demands. In Dax's situation the two realms of physical existence that usually interweave are divided. His own overwhelming reality is embodiment, while his therapists, in their relation to him, are disembodied.

The phenomenon of pain per se cannot account for the drastic bodily dichotomy between Dax and his therapists. Other factors are involved. First, the therapists' actions are the cause of the treatment and its pain, and those actions are performed without Dax's permission. In addition, he is physically powerless to resist, to flee, or even to shield his body. Finally, familiar avenues—the eyes and the hands—that lead out of the body and away from its pain are permanently closed.

The first of these, the causing of pain and the absence of consent, will be discussed in the context of moral views; because they call immediately for an interpretive moral framework, there can be no validity in discussing them purely phenomenologically. But the other factors, physical helplessness and the virtual loss of hands and eyes, are not in themselves moral problems. They create a situation of altered embodiment that is prior to, and in Dax's case a condition for, morally problematic treatment. Their discussion therefore belongs here, since they by themselves, even without the added experience of pain, are sufficient to generate a serious existential—and eventually moral—gulf between Dax and his therapists.

The eyes and hands are the two senses, as it were, with the most developed duality of receiving the world as well as entering and altering it. Vision can passively register everything available, as well as actively select, frame, and edit. Between persons the eyes become still more powerful, able to intrude as well as to deflect intrusion. The hands are the material version of this almost metaphysical power of vision. Through touch they receive the world's physical reality, and through the wielding of tools they remake it. The hand, itself the original tool and still the supreme one for many tasks, symbolizes as does no other part of the body the power of reconstructing the world for human purposes. Together, eyes and hands represent freedom from the body's monopoly. Without them, until other capacities can be developed in their place, the only parameter of existence is embodiment. The ease of outreaching the body and taking on the world is lost; within its boundaries the body becomes all-powerful, while against external reality it is helpless.

In Dax's case helplessness is emphasized by the phenomenon of prolonged nakedness. The result is an intensely paradoxical experience combining the exteriority of forced openness and the closed isolation of an interiority without eyes or hands. Singly, these conditions might not be insurmountable. Naked, he could fend off others' gazes with his eyes, were he sighted. Blind, he could hide from other eyes, were he capable of covering his nakedness. But naked, blind, and helpless, he is wholly submerged in the body. For others too, his body is his very being, fully exposed to them, unprotected and public, stripped in some places even of its skin.

For himself and for his therapists, Dax's existence is defined by the body. But, unlike him, they are disembodied. "The one with authority and power has no body for his inferiors. He cannot, for example, be seen without clothing."[3] In Dax's situation—in clinical situations generally—the discrepancy between the hidden body of the therapist and the exposed, emphasized body of the patient is not an outward sign of the distance between them; it is a source of that distance. Dax's therapists cannot be seen with or without their clothing, since in his case they cannot be seen at all, while he cannot be unseen. Nor can he feel their bodies, clasp their hands in his. They touch him at their discretion, usually gloved and with instruments, reminding him palpably of his own body more than theirs. In every respect, his embodiment is intensified to the highest degree, while theirs is omitted entirely from their relationship to him. They are voices with tools but not bodies.

The power their tools represent, the power of overcoming not only the body's limits but the given forms of the world, increases the discrepancy between their disembodiment and Dax. Without tools, he has no means of physically altering his world. Exactly because of his inability, he provides to others almost unlimited possibility in that regard through their reconstruction of his body. That which is forbidden to him is their freedom, the escape from embodiment through making, remaking, affecting the world. The destruction of that possibility in him directly increases it for them. His loss is their gain because he is their gain; it is his body through which they transcend their own. The remaking of the human body can be considered the supreme artifice, but though he provides the material for that ultimate recreating, it is a project in which he cannot participate.[4] From their point of view, it would be better were he not even present consciously; his pain and protests interfere. From his therapists the work of artifice demands the most concentrated sentience; from him, only nonsentience that submits like a stone to the sculptor.

The chasm between Dax's body and his therapists' disembodiment is not an anomaly owed to external features of his situation. It is intrinsic to the experience of being burned, blinded, helpless, and repeatedly reconstructed. For both sides the gulf is inevitable; overpowering embodiment and disembodiment entail one another. But though inevitable, the chasm is not yet unbridgeable; only moral certainty can make it so.

In turning now to moral frameworks, which are essential to invoke the moment pain is knowingly inflicted, it will soon be clear that the wider the existential chasm becomes, the more hopelessly uninhabitable will be the moral structures erected on either side of it. For that reason it will be important to return, in the final section, to the gulf between embodiment and disembodiment to consider how it may be crossed, even—and especially—when pain is present.

III

The causing of pain is the antithesis of medicine, friendship, and parenting—the forms of caring represented in the group advocating treatment for Dax. Of these, medicine in particular is concerned explicitly with the prevention and the relief of pain. Friends and parents, less typically in a therapeutic role, at least are concerned not to cause pain. That any of these should be responsible for deliberate action that is known to produce pain is incomprehensible within the commitments just outlined. For both the one who inflicts pain and the one who suffers, it is urgent that those commitments be reinterpreted in order to make sense of their violation. The alternative is moral chaos, a condition that may serve in less-demanding circumstances but cannot suffice in a state of moral emergency like Dax's.

Pain constitutes a moral emergency when it cannot be reconciled with the motives an individual has supposed to be present. The surrender to chaos in that case is the conclusion that there are no discoverable intentions behind the pain, that the natural world is indifferent to human life, just as other human life is indifferent to one's own. This view may serve to patch the occasional tear in an otherwise intact fabric. But a complete garment of moral belief cannot be patterned after indifference, since it is the very negation of humanly meaningful pattern. Some intention has to be trusted. Even evil motives are more human, more bearable, than the chaos of cosmic indifference.

Neither Dax nor his therapists can survive days and months of pain without belief in an intention behind it. In what motive are they to believe? Do his therapists, in short, intend him harm or good? The question is not an empirical one but an inquiry about which moral belief to hold when harm and good seem inverted, when life is refused by Dax as though a harm, pain advocated by his therapists as though a good. In what moral frameworks are these inversions intelligible?

The two structures of moral belief that accommodate most unambiguously the inflicting of pain are political torture and divine beneficence. For Dax and his therapists, representing two sides struggling to bring moral order into a situation of inflicted pain, the possibilities open to them are interpretation of the pain as governed by evil motive or good.

In torture, pain is experienced as unequivocally evil because only harm, and unlimited harm, is intended by it. The fact that a regime claims to legitimize the pain in terms of a political good is unrelated to the evil that the person experiences it to be. The effectiveness of torture in fact depends upon the unambiguous character of pain to defeat the individual and produce the desired confession or·information. If the pain could be identified even remotely with good in the victim's view, it could be longer endured, as comparable suffering may be endured, for example, in combat. Withholding the "betrayal" desired by the regime is not a sufficient good to redeem the pain, since often there is no information to be given, no confession that would be accepted. The pain inflicted in torture is an unqualified evil for its victim because it is intended to be so, the destruction of an individual—and perhaps reconstruction—for the captors' ends.

Is the moral structure of torture analogous to Dax's situation as he, or his therapists, might experience it? Specifically, is the end which his pain is intended to serve an end that Dax himself regards as a good, or is it a good only in the view of his therapists? Does his pain, in short, serve others' interests or his own?

Viewing his therapists' intention as political and Dax as their victim is of course extreme, for it inflates one element—force—into an overall framework. Again, however, the question is not empirical validity but coherence as a moral structure in which pain can be understood unambiguously. In that, the framework succeeds. All that it involves is that Dax, in sincere and sound mind, believes that his therapists recognize their intentions to be unrelated to his good, that is, unrelated to his precise, personally defined, concrete interest.

That lack of relation they do recognize. The good they intend is in the direction of different ends, abstract and impersonal: an undefined future Dax, an ideal of rehabilitation, a devotion to Life. These are the values of the regime, the ideology which Dax's pain is to serve. His individual good is not identified. He himself is barely known to them, and then only negatively, in terms of what he is not or of what he is like (and thus is not): "You're like a marathon runner. . . ." "If you're the man I've been led to believe you are. . . ." "He wasn't going to be Don Cowart anymore." Then who was he going to be? And who will he be in the meantime? No one asks. Only one thing is known about the present person; he refuses the goals of the therapists. The good they intend, unrelated to him, benefits him only if he renounces his heresy. The purpose of the pain is not his confession but his conversion. "We do not destroy the heretic because he resists us; so long as he resists us we never destroy him. We convert him, we capture his inner mind, we reshape him. We burn all evil and all illusion out of him; we bring him over to our side." [5]

Dax's refusal to consent to the pain, his powerlessness to escape, and the absence of a recognized relation between his good and the goals of his therapists are basis enough for a comparison with torture. But a more basic parallel exists, without which the inflicting of pain would be impossible. That is the chasm already described between one whose embodiment is intensified beyond bearing and one who is "so without any human recognition of or identification with the pain that he is not only able to bear its presence but able to bring it continually into the present, inflict it, sustain it, minute after minute, hour after hour." [6] The inflicting of pain for any purpose requires dissociation from one's own body in order not to suffer with the person in pain. The relief that dissociation affords accounts for the experience in which it can be easier to intervene in someone's pain by increasing it (as in child battering) than simply to witness it and suffer in response. Causing pain in another becomes a means of preventing it in oneself, because in deliberately inflicting it on another, a decisive repudiation of one's own body is accomplished. In circumstances where much suffering is witnessed and much inflicted, eliminating the possibility of the agent's pain is a prerequisite. If, in addition, the circumstances involve caring, as does clinical work, this adds the requirement that the agent, the carer, be able to say "I know that it hurts" without being able to mean it.

The chasm that disembodiment can create in clinical situations may be greater than is needed even for torture. Precisely because therapists want to comfort, as the torturer does not, they court the possibility of their own pain, of crossing the chasm in an unguarded moment. That danger must be removed to make sympathy practical. They must be categorically safe from suffering in order to venture even verbally across the distance between themselves and someone in pain. Their safety comes from motive, from the urgency and worthiness of the good that is served. Their voices calling over the chasm to Dax appeal insistently to that good, reminding themselves more than him why they can neither join him in his suffering nor release him from it. But the distance maintained to accommodate caring can as easily accommodate torture, if the good they represent is as fraudulent to him as the torturer's motive is to the prisoner. Like the treatment tub that seems to promise comfort and cradling but instead holds searing chemicals, the verbal expressions of caring themselves become sources of pain when they parody caring; they are worse than silence. They remind him that the voices, though they be right at his ear, come from no one's lips, come—like the voice of a bodiless god—from an infinite distance that he cannot bridge.

IV

The comparison of Dax's suffering with torture provides a morally unambiguous reading of his experience. As an extreme view, its instability is due not to a lack of congruence with the situation, but to the tendency of an extreme to evoke its opposite, even turn into its opposite, in this case beneficence. That instability would prevail and ambiguity be daily rekindled unless one or the other of the views is maintained with almost fanatic adherence.

The moral structure of torture readily suggests its opposite. Only a god could intend a purely transcendent good, unrelated to individuals. Only a god could be truly without body, incapable of suffering. But would a god want to create pain? If we view Dax's therapists as representing not an evil regime but an omnipotent Good, we must locate the place of pain in the framework of divine beneficence: why would a supreme power, capable of infinite blessing and bounty, inflict suffering?

Two customary explanations must be dismissed first. One is that such a being does not cause pain but allows it to occur through other agents or through chance. This is a reformulation, not a dilution, of causality. It fails to remove responsibility for pain from a supreme power, since an omnipotent being is the agent, directly or indirectly, of all that occurs. A limited god might leave some outcomes to chance, but they would then forever be inexplicable, ambiguous at best, evidence of incompetence at worst. In Dax's situation ambiguity is the problem that a moral framework is required to solve and therefore cannot count as a solution. Worse, a view in which pain is the result of incompetence is tantamount to a belief in cosmic indifference, a useless view in a state of moral emergency. If the limited power of gods or of therapists is offered to explain Dax's pain, nothing is gained, for the invoking of limitations—human or divine—can be used to excuse flawed beneficence, even evil intention, as easily as failed power. And if beneficence cannot be relied upon, a moral structure based upon it collapses.

The second familiar answer to the problem of why a purely good being might inflict pain is punishment. But punishment is a practice to which only finite beings resort, who can find no other means of expressing disapproval or no other form of relief except retaliation. The permutations of pain and punishment in the human imagination are beyond the scope of this discussion; the point that is relevant here is simply that punishment is evidence of failure, not of the offender but of the offended. Thus, it looms large in the human repertoire of pain giving but has no place in the divine.

For what other motive would pain be inflicted by a being of perfect power and beneficence? For a god without limitations and thus without physical form, the greatest obstacle for believers is the seeming unreality of one who permanently eludes perception. Creatures for whom the body is the ground of existence must be able to maintain belief in a bodiless power whose evidence of existence is at most a voice. Their belief, when it wavers, can be restored in only one way. They must reencounter the power they have doubted. Since a spiritual being cannot materially appear before them in order to dispel their doubts, the experience of their own bodies has to serve as verification. The most intense of the body's experiences is pain; it is through the inflicting of pain, therefore, that the inexperienceable affirms its existence, that "the incontestable reality of the sensory world becomes the incontestable reality of a world invisible and unable to be touched."[7] Pain is neither punishment, correction, nor a chance side effect. It is a display of power, but not for the pleasure of overpowering or the pride of display. Its purpose is solely to make blessing possible by renewing the belief through which all blessing comes.

Other, benign, expressions of power would not achieve this. They instead would have the effect of alleviating embodiment; the effect of material bounty is to become free of the body's tyranny, to approach disembodiment, to suppose oneself a god rather than a creature in need of one. The effect of pain is the opposite, to remove doubt by restoring true belief, the belief that a real god exists. Not all pain serves this purpose, of course; not the suffering that is part of mundane existence, but that which is unmistakably directed against wavering belief: pain that is distinctly, dramatically, wounding. Only that suffering confirms to despairing believers that infinite power and goodness exist. "Unable to apprehend God with conviction, they will—after the arrival of the plague or the disease-laden quail or the fire or the sword or the storm—apprehend him in the intensity of the pain in their own bodies."[8]

Can Dax and his therapists be understood in this framework? Is it plausible to interpret his pain as a renewal of belief in beneficence?

Dax experiences, in addition to the lingering hurt of the original injury, the wounding pain caused by his therapists as they heal him. He cannot see them; they are only voices. But even could he observe them, he never would glimpse the force whereby they work their healing changes within him. That force of healing, the therapists' power to bless, cannot itself be apprehended. For Dax, however, the failure to believe in it would be fatal. To doubt its existence and turn from his benefactors would mean his destruction. Only the pain they are able to inflict can affirm for him their power to bless; the intransigence of his doubt is but evidence of his need for continuing affirmation to save him from the delusion that death is preferable.

The place of wounding in beneficence is not a comfortable

moral view. We are more familiar with perversions of it that make of beneficence a farce: a parent insisting "I am hurting you because I love you," or wounding heralded as a trial and temptation, a divine test of belief. Surely it would be monstrous to propose that Dax's therapists hurt him because they can find no better way to communicate their caring, or that they inflict pain to reassure themselves of his faith in them. In true beneficence he is hurt, not as a deformed intention of good, but solely in order to make possible his receiving the blessing available, the healing that he must have to live. Nor is the pain an entrapment to try his belief by giving him reason for doubt; it is instead a reason for belief, a means of apprehending the power in which it is lifesaving to believe.

V

Making moral sense of Dax's pain by either interpretation, beneficence or torture, is a costly means of resolving ambiguity. Both frameworks succeed in dispelling confusion about the intention behind his pain, but at the price of distancing the two sides so extremely that ambiguity is clarified into antagonism and moral uncertainty becomes a fight to the death. In either framework, refusal of the powerless side to submit will result in its annihilation. But the antagonism and ensuing death struggle between victim and torturer, between doubt and beneficence, can occur only in a situation already characterized by an existential abyss like that described between patient and therapist. Having seen the extremity, then, to which moral understanding is driven in situations predicated on that gulf, we must return to it now and consider how it might be crossed.

In torture and in beneficence power flows in one direction. Similarly in Dax's case, voices and instruments cross the gulf from one side, the therapists'. But unilateral power widens the gap rather than closing it. The actions of reaching across are not ways of joining him in embodiment; they are signals from a realm of agency where the body is insignificant. For an actual crossing to occur, two changes are necessary. He must be assisted to reach beyond the imprisoning body, while they must find ways of reinhabiting their own bodies in relation to his. Each must, in short, move genuinely in the direction of the other.

Dax has no physical means of extending himself beyond the body, but he has—like his therapists—a voice. He is capable of articulate speech, reasoned argument, self-description. The voice is his form of self-extension; speech, his instrument for altering his world; refusal, his weapon. The degree of injury he inflicts by his rejection of treatment can be measured in the wounded cry from the other side, "Then why am I in medicine?"

His voice is a projection of self beyond body and suffering because it is more than a scream of agony, more than an audible form of the body's recoil without content that could engage a listener. His is not the formless protest of sufferers whose cries only frustrate their hearers. "Devoid of any content other than complaint, their utterances are self-trivializing and dissolute, a form of inarticulate pre-language that carries no power to legitimize their suffering, their hunger, their fear, their doubt, their exhaustion, or to legitimize our notice of these things. If their voices were able to form and express these things, the story would be a different story."[9] Dax's *is* a different story. His voice is not dismissible. It reaches across the chasm to grip his listeners in a dialogue that becomes the beginning of a bridge between them, an engagement from which neither side releases the other.

The transcending of embodiment through speech would be possible even if Dax were without words, provided that someone spoke, as it were, with his voice, legitimizing his claims by giving them the power of language to engage others. That is possible only when the other voice arises, like the claims themselves, from the depths of embodiment. He cannot be represented by the language of bodiless advocates. This, then, raises the second concern, mirroring Dax's need for extension beyond the body: the need for his therapists to transcend disembodiment, to experience the world from within the body as he does. How is that more substantial spanning of the gulf between them to be achieved, the flying buttress without which the arch of their voices finally must fall?

The task is to uncover to Dax their embodiment. Since it is not the fact but the meanings of having a body that their disembodiment denies, literal disclosure of the body misses the point. Clinical practices that mimic self-disclosure—professionals shedding official garb, sitting on the patient's bed, letting patients examine them—fail for that reason. Far from divulging personal meanings of embodiment, they are an exercise in disembodiment, a display of the extent to which the body's facticity can be bared without the person "inside" being forced out. The practices are not without risk since they flirt with embodiment, but they are a gratuitous flirting, freely initiated, freely ended, unlike the patient's embodiment. When the daring goes too far and a person is caught, shame arises from exposure not of the body but of the game, a trivial charade performed in the face of the patient's genuine, unfree embodiment.

While Dax's sightlessness makes literal for him the disembodied state of his therapists, recovery of sight would not alter that state, just as professional familiarity toward patients proves to them no more than is known already, namely, the fact of a body's existence. The proof of embodiment comes not through seeing or touching a body but through experiencing its implications. Thus it would be no more conclusive for his therapists verbally to disclose to Dax their hunger, fatigue, or other interior states than for them visibly to disclose their bodies to him, were that possible. He requires different evidence, evidence that the body has a significant bearing on their lives.

How is the significance of the body to be conveyed? How is he to discover that they too are embodied? One means is by their revealing to him the vulnerability that summarizes for them, as for him, the body's implications, disclosing to him their bewilderment, anguish, incomprehension, fear. It is the attempt at disembodiment that has made these phenomena seem like purely psychological states, unrelated to physical experience, when in fact their origin lies in the limitations inherent in the body. A bodiless being is invulnerable, at least to the forms of destruction that we know. Vulnerability manifested willingly by one person to another is thus a testimony to the significance of embodiment.

A second testimony, enlarging infinitely upon the first, is the transmuting of vulnerability into its opposite, the power to allay it. From that transmuting emerge an intensity of empathic regard and a corresponding refinement of physical ministration in which the smallest gesture, the least touch, is capable of easing the other's suffering. In that ministration is found the positive pole in the dynamic of embodiment, the fact that vulnerability itself is vulnerable. Even at its worst it can be assuaged, but only through the forms of caring that an empathic—because embodied—imagination creates.

Bridging the chasm in these ways removes none of the moral ambiguity about the motive for Dax's pain. But it relieves the urgency for erecting moral structures in which to anchor pain and its motive. In a situation composed strictly of one side unilaterally acting upon the other, motives are crucial. They lose their importance in reciprocal action in which the disparity between two sides is continually overcome as each extends itself across the gulf toward the other. The fact that his therapists inflict pain and Dax experiences it describes one layer of their reality. But beyond that, he is able to project himself outside the torment of embodiment, and they in turn are able to emerge from disembodiment. Their bodies as well as their voices answer his voice and body.

As long as they and he remain mutually engaged in each other's vulnerability and its alleviation, the existential distance between them diminishes, and with it the chasm on which are predicated both torture and beneficence. The moment that mutuality is abandoned and the chasm reopened, then power is again unilateral, pain again a moral emergency, and each side must take refuge in one extreme view or the other. The difference between the views disappears beside the dark fact that in both the chasm becomes finally unbridgeable. In either framework, beneficence or torture, an existential disparity that in itself is ever amenable to softening, hardens into moral clarity, into an antagonism sharp and intractable. That antagonism removes from pain any confusion about its motive as well as any means of its alleviation. A decade into Dax's story neither side has silenced the other or erased the pain's ambiguity. The years have not proved either side right. Instead, perhaps Dax and his therapists have concluded that preserving a bridge between them for as many decades as pain is remembered matters more than moral certainty.

NOTES

1. Elaine Scarry, *The Body in Pain: The Making and Unmaking of the World* (New York: Oxford University Press, 1985), 152.

2. Ibid., 47, 276.

3. Ibid., 210.

4. Ibid., 253.

5. George Orwell, *1984* (New York: The New American Library, Inc., 1983), 210.

6. Scarry, *The Body in Pain*, 36.

7. Ibid., 202.

8. Ibid., 201.

9. Ibid.

On Why We Should Not Agree with Dax ▨ *Stanley Johannesen*

THE FILM *DAX'S CASE* IS ABOUT A MAN WHO HAS A quarrel with us. Dax's "case," to use the word in its colloquial sense as a feeling of grievance, a gripe, is that he ought to have been allowed to die. Not now, not any longer, but at some point in the past during the treatment of his injuries and in other periods of intense physical and mental suffering that were the outcome of his injuries. There have been other notable instances of people wishing to die, or wishing to have assistance in dying, because of their sufferings, or because of the prospect of utterly hopeless existence. Dax's case is unusual in that even with the return of a degree of hopefulness, and even success (both worldly success in the usual terms, and limited and circumscribed success in living with his manifold handicaps), Dax wants still to make his point, to carry his case, retrospectively. He makes a claim on us, in other words, which is in addition to whatever he has successfully claimed by means of legal processes and by exploiting the means to personal fulfillment open to everyone in our society. He wants us to agree with him that he ought to have been allowed to die.

It is important that we make sense of this claim, and important that we recognize the complex and difficult sort of claim that it is. It is complex and difficult in part because of the complexity and difficulty of unravelling the story—of establishing the facts, crediting recollections worn smooth with retelling, sorting out the impossible issues of self-interest and self-protection, and so forth. There is in Dax Cowart's story a compelling human drama, of decent and troubled people acting in uncharted territory with sometimes conflicting guiding principles, and with the tendencies of all of us to see our past actions through the simplifying lenses of what we suppose to be the lessons we have learned.

There is another sense, however, in which the complexity and difficulty of Dax's claim has rather less to do with establishing harmony and balance in the tellers' accounts of their experiences and rather more to do with establishing in ourselves, as hearers and beholders, a secure ground for whatever response we make. To hear the claim of another that he ought to have been allowed to die—that is, to hear it as a valid moral claim on ourselves—is to experience a peculiar and powerful claim on the limits of social responsibility, on collective membership. A traditional formula that expresses what we usually recognize as the limits of collective membership and responsibility for one another is "life, liberty and the pursuit of happiness." The right to die, if one may so put the implied claim in its civic dimension, lifts the social contract out of its classical context of sociability altogether and puts it in a much more modern and radically individualistic context. Dax's case, seen in this light, exposes far more than our capacities as beholders for sentimental identification with suffering; it also exposes the stresses to which sociability has been put in our civic and social traditions. What I want to do in this essay is to suggest some of the ways Dax troubles us as beholders, what we owe him, and what we owe to ourselves.

I

Let us be clear about the affecting power of Dax Cowart's story: Our response to the demand of an injured person that he ought to have been allowed to die, even that he had a right to die, is not based on a fully empathetic entry into his private experience. Or rather, we cannot both enter into his experience and attend to his claims. To enter his experience is to be blind, to have the memory of specific pain, to have evolved a personality anguished by feelings of helplessness, despair, and persecution over long periods of time. Few of us should claim we can know such a story in other than the most conventionalized and sentimental terms.

On the other hand, unless we are competent members of our social and material worlds in precisely the ways that make it impossible for us to empathize with Dax Cowart, we cannot attend to him at all. Claims about the fundamental injustice of arrangements we normally approve of require dispassion. Claims about states of affairs that have to be seen to be evaluated require that we have eyes to see, that we be very much unlike Dax Cowart. So much is implicit in the choice of the medium of film, and in the voyeurist conception of moral realism in which film traditions stand. There is, in short, a curious symmetry of incompetence on either side of the divide of experience and representation in the telling and hearing of Dax's story. His need, and ours, is to reach agreement. Yet Dax's experience is closed to us, and ours is closed to him.

Our religious and civic practices exist in part to mediate telling and listening, showing and beholding, across the chasm of personal incompetence. In Michael Ignatieff's interesting phrases, the decent society takes the language of individual wants and demands, and by means of translation through its accumulated moral experience, turns it into an understanding of legitimate "needs"—even when the unmediated language of "wants" is immoderate, unfulfillable, perhaps incomprehensible.[1] Another way of putting it would be to say that the responsibility of society, through its religious and civic practices, is to effect, when faced with radical incompetence in knowing the experience of others or in interpreting their wants, an upward displacement of moral bonds to whatever level is necessary in order to restore understanding. In religion this is grace, or beatitude; in civic life it is justice.

The case of Dax Cowart is exquisitely rich in opportunity for reflection on these issues. Dax wants to die. But what does he need? How will we know what this is? Which of our collective practices will allow us to displace this problem into a moral plane that allows both Dax and us membership of a whole, whether in grace or justice? The documentary film is indeed one of our practices, and *Dax's Case* is an effort to move us toward comprehension, and even toward grace and justice, along an axis of interpretation having to do with Dax's treatment by his doctors and Dax's attempts to assert a particular right—the right to die as he chooses. Now the language of rights is, so to speak, the intrinsic idiom of the documentary film. It is an affinity forged in a particular culture, with a particular sense of political rights and of the use of practices of realism in safeguarding those rights. Our question here, however, is this: Is the language of rights the place we want to end up in? Are we sure we can take this up in good faith on these terms? Or, to begin with a simpler question: What is Dax's case about anyway?

II

Profound disfigurement aborts many of the common and reassuring signals by means of which ordinary life is conducted between people. It commonly effects a serious transgression of rules concerning ritual and social pollution. Of the sons of Aaron, the progenitor of the priestly caste among the ancient Hebrews, any of them who was, among other things, "broken-footed, or broken-handed, or crook-backed, or a dwarf, or that hath a blemish in his eye, or is scurvy, or scabbed, or hath his stones broken" was forbidden by Yahweh to "come nigh unto the altar, because he hath a blemish; that he profane not my sanctuaries" (Leviticus 21:16–23). This ritual disability did not extend so far into social practice as to license cruelty and ostracism: The sacred writer notes that disfigured priests were nonetheless to "eat the bread of their God"—that is, to subsist on the Temple practice.

This fastidious ritual prohibition of the Hebrews is by no means the most cruel reaction to disfigurement of which human societies are capable. The impulse here is perhaps something rather nearer the opposite of cruelty. If we allow, in an unsentimental view of human nature, that a natural symbolism biased toward symmetry, predictability, and the golden mean is an inescapable part of the apparatus of human feeling, then it is a triumph of culture, of the artificial structure of highly developed human social bonds, that these reactions against disfigurement and damaged persons are contained by regulation, by a rule of law. The striking feature of the Hebrew law governing the Aaronic priesthood is, in this perspective, not that blemished individuals were prohibited from participating in the cultic practices of the Temple. After all, these rites were in themselves just such affirmations of regularity, harmony, principles of magical compensation, and substitutionary enactment as would have to disappear if blemish and irregularity were tolerated in their precincts. That blemished members of the priestly order were nonetheless permitted to live on the workings of the Temple cult suggests what is more crucial to the Hebrew social order: namely, an understanding that ethical norms, unlike ritual norms, must take into account an additional factor. An element of compassion, an ability to "feel with," shoulders aside the demands of natural symbolism at just that point where the law remarks the transition from ritual to ordinary life. Since the law allows for feeling on both sides of this divide, for purity *and* compassion, there is no dangerous repression of feeling on this question, nor is there danger of confusing ritual necessity with the real world.

The danger of confusing the ideal with the real is nowhere better illustrated in modern history than in the German genocidal war against the Jews. The "Nazi biomedical vision," as Robert Jay Lifton calls it, fused elements of German national myth and traditional anti-Semitism, on the one hand, with elements of modern sanitary-disposal engineering, on the other, to create a unique but terrifyingly human horror.[2] As Lifton points out, once the separation of racial fantasy from social reality was bridged by ideology and law in a modern state, not even the professional ethics and traditional compassion of the practice of medicine was proof against the profoundest perversion of feeling. On the contrary, medicine itself provided the metaphors and the techniques by means of which mass murder could seem the restoration of health: therapeutic surgery applied to the body of the nation. What was eventually applied to the extermination of Jews was begun in Germany by experiments on the insane, the ill, and the unfit. The Germans, in other words, might be said to have lacked what is implicit in the Mosaic code governing blemished priests, a way to recognize and institutionalize human bonds in such a way as to place them beyond the operations of the tribal or the national cult. Lacking this capacity, a modern society is peculiarly vulnerable to obsessions with efficiency, consistency, and thoroughness; in short, to an obsession with the pseudoscientific.

The example of Nazi Germany so haunts the modern consciousness we are perhaps sometimes in danger of overlooking something else, something equally instructive in the case of the blemished priests: namely the provision for the ritual channeling of otherwise repressed feelings of revulsion. The film *Dax's Case* supplies material for meditation across the whole field of feelings about blemished and damaged human existence, not least because it exhibits a typical modern confusion as to exactly what the central moral issue is. There is no escaping, for example, in the nature of Dax's complaint of his treatment, in the way that the film follows a narrative line in and out of these episodes of treatment, and in the way that a succession of medical practitioners willingly assumes moral responsibility for the consequences of their several professional acts, that the film is meant to make of the systematized, efficient, mechanized, pragmatic, and experimental ethos of contemporary medical practice a kind of moral warning. Medical treatment itself, the film seems to say, is the probable point of entry, however conscientious or well-meaning its practitioners, into a social nightmare of forced dehumanization. Dax himself has little doubt of this. The images of imprisonment and of tortures by unwanted treatment that dominate his own recollection of his experience speak eloquently of a pervasive unease in our culture with the technological sophistication and impersonality of modern medicine. It seems doubtful, however, that these harsh images, understandable in Dax's extremely traumatized physical and mental state, would also resonate throughout our deepest personal and collective fears of the future were it not for the Nazi experience. We are right, on the basis of that experience, to question closely any submission of human life to automatic processes, whether technological or bureaucratic. The profoundest evil comes on the cat feet of duty, routine, plausibility.

Yet it must be said that if this is the sole, or even major, lesson to derive from Dax's experiences, the case fits awkwardly the lesson it is meant to reinforce. Dax's doctors are manifestly civilized and deeply humane men; Dax was not caught in a systematic sweep of victims of ideology, nor was he selected at random for medical experiments. It is not the doctors in this cautionary tale who are groping for a rationale for death in terms of a political myth, but Dax himself—in the view that in the United States a person should be able to do whatever he or she wants.

A curious consequence of attending to the wrong lesson in this event may be to fail to notice what side of things we are ending up on, and for what reasons. If we are persuaded by a film that a badly injured young man ought to have been allowed to die when he wanted to, we are either influenced by his political ideology and do not need the visual evidence of his tragedy, or we need the visual evidence and are therefore calling our repressed revulsion into play to assent to a death that would otherwise seem unnecessary as a premature and wasteful death. The disturbing thing about this other "message" of the episode in the film is that the feeling of revulsion, which is patently capitalized on for purposes of assent to the justice of Dax's demand, is unacknowledged. The beholder is not allowed a choice in terms of this natural reaction, nor is Dax permitted full membership in a healthy society, one that not only respects rights, but also releases its feelings in appropriate contexts and rituals. I should like to make a case here for the proposition that the *social* tragedy of Dax's life was not the system that treated him against his will, but the one that supplied him with no other language than the language of "rights," and no other claim on his fellows than that he be allowed to die.

III

One must assume that to assent to the death of another as a good, as a social good, as a good productive of worthy collective ends, is to have in mind the appropriate ritual for that death. Death without ritual is monstrous, a sort of garbage disposal, wholly repugnant both to the Hellenistic bases of our civilization, in which body is character, and to the Hebrew and Christian tradition of the final exhumation of all flesh. As public witnesses to the exposure of Dax's body in treatment, a scene medieval in its graphic horror, we are parties to a certain reversal of the appropriate order of ritual. In the appropriate order of ritual, the body of the dead becomes a public property, and public sentiment and practices determine how the corpse is disposed of. Above all, the appearance of the corpse in death is attributed to the operations of death itself, personified as a man or thing who is the last enemy—as the grim reaper, and so forth. Public ritual wages the victorious war that the individual always fails to win. Death is swallowed up in victory in the anticipation of the last trump when the dead will rise with new bodies.

The shock of the encounter with Dax's body is that while the appearance is that of a corpse, the body is not yet a public property; it belongs to a living man. Instead of the public realm claiming the corpse for a ritual enactment of triumph over death, the public realm is accused in this film of keeping control of this body away from its owner, the individual person whose body it is. That person says he wants to be allowed to die, but not in the traditional sense— that is, to submit to the surrender of his body to the public realm of ritual and myth—but as a political act of separation from public authority.

The issues here are complex, and must be teased out with great deliberation. Already one must flag a disturbing implication of this reversal of affect toward the public realm. A public whose sentiments are prepared to endorse a wish to die, in retrospect, and on account of a sentimental revulsion to the appearance of death in the living, without at the same time having prepared for the ritual enactment of that death, has abandoned all its members to the most lonely sort of death, a death in which there is no struggle and eventual triumph, but only the net implications of evidences of morbidity, and a certain pity which is repressed revulsion. If the body in our society is no longer the site of a struggle between the enemy—which is death—and the public purpose—which is civic and celestial immortality—what is it then? Of what is it the sign? Dax's case is profoundly instructive.

Dax's body presents itself to us in the film, as befits the productions of a business civilization, as itself a product. The image of Dax's body shows us that something went terribly wrong with an industrial process and a business that should be able to deliver better products if it is going to deliver them at all. The argument is not specifically that the medical business was capable of delivering a better product than it did in Dax's case during the 1970s, but rather that knowing that it could not do any better it should not have delivered the faulty product that it did—that is, Dax's pain-wracked and deformed body. This is perhaps too harsh a way to put the case, but it really only very slightly alters the images and language of the principals themselves, and it permits us to see how some equally plausible narratives might have been constructed from this episode.

Unwanted products, in a business view of things, are equivalent to a cost of doing business. If we are to follow the logic of the film's scrutiny of the medical business, and say that Dax's body is too high a cost for whatever advance in medical resources resulted from treating him, then we should pursue this question of costs back into the accident that began it all. It becomes at once clear that the idea of an "accident" is purely ideological. The laying of pipelines full of highly volatile products, like many other actions in the course of doing business, has attached to it a cost in terms of burnt bodies, of permanently altered flesh. Altered bodies are not a wanted product of such activities, but they are a product. However statistically small the occurrence of these products, they are unavoidable and therefore in a sense necessary. What is necessary in business, such as security systems, industrial spies, and tax accountants, cannot be said to be unproductive, although there is a powerful tradition of economic thought that denies this.[3] If we are only barely able to grasp the necessary in these business activities, how much more difficulty do we experience in accepting the necessity of burnt bodies?

Consider whether we would feel as fully the force of Dax's case had he been burned in combat, had he been burned by his own carelessness, or in the course of criminal activity. In the latter cases the "cost" would have been a cost to Dax of his own folly; in the former case the "cost" would have been a prefigured cost of waging war, a cost chargeable to the war-making rationality which has a solid and unembarrassed legitimacy in our society.[4] "Accident," in the tradition of the capitalist workplace, operates to cut off a similar analysis. Dax's injuries were nonetheless a "cost" of economic organization and commercial activity, prefigured in insurance rates and budgetary allowances for legal defense fees, but not socially acknowledged. When something is necessary but unacknowledged, it is likely to produce an irrational reaction, a search for a place to discharge frustration and anger. Is it possible that our focus on the medical business as the place where something went wrong is a diversion from attention to a process that we cannot or will not scrutinize, much less openly accept and defend? Stripped in advance of its status as a cost of doing business, Dax's body is reinterpreted as a product of healing institutions and practices and the cost is sentimentally carried to Dax's interior. Dax's interior, the ghost in the machine, pays the cost in suffering for the product of the healing institution which is his new body.

Our culture has distinctive and extremely stubborn resistances to pursuing justice, except in such sentimental terms as to make the receipt of justice hollow, lonely, and terrible. To be sure, Dax was paid an immense sum out of court for his pains. It is, however, characteristic of our sentimental principles that this compensation is only slyly winked at in the film, and in any case cannot be held to have anything to do with the sentimental issues. The gift of money is as unrealized ritually as is the mortification of Dax's flesh. The argument here is not that in our documentary realism we should prefer to shove our inquisitorial microphones and lenses in the faces of oil-company executives and their lawyers instead of in the faces of doctors. The argument is that a society with the means for compensating people with huge sums of money is not absolved of the responsibility for giving that money, as it should give its medical care, in love, with the open and acknowledged gift of ritual compensation and membership. Has Dax received all that we can give him out of our spiritual resources if we agree that being damaged as he was he ought to have been allowed to die?

IV

Consider the sort of sign that Dax's body has become for us when it is taken to be the outcome of an accident and of unwanted treatment. We turn again to notice how the traditional emblem of the corpse signified something grand, in which revulsion and inevitability were both acknowledged, but both transcended. Dax's body is visually now a piece of public property but as it is it cannot symbolize anything in the traditional sense. We do not personify death. Nor do we care for the soul in the flesh except sentimentally—that is, as something that does not survive beyond the state of our own feelings about it, feelings which in any case are not openly acknowledged. Dax's body is not a natural metaphor for us. It does not for us naturally and without special effort resemble a condition, moral or political, that we are prepared freely to substitute in our discourse for the symbol of his body. We reserve for such functions the symbol of the whole and healthy body. The athlete, the beautiful youth, the vigorous champion, resemble and may therefore be said to symbolize our thought about the social body. A broken body, rich as it may be in the symbology of Christian faith, does not, in a dechristianized world, symbolize anything by resembling it. As a sign, the broken body is therefore something of an index or an indicator. An indicator does not resemble the thing indicated or stand as a substitute for that thing, but instead shows where in the general scheme of things it is to be found. An indicator marks the site of an event. One might say that Dax's body stands to the condition of thought in our culture about moral obligation, as the Turin shroud stands to a certain condition of Christian piety. In each case the thing retains marks of a lost image, marks that are no more than stains, blemishes that are not the images themselves, but mark the site of a damage, indexes to the extent of a wound. Both are liable to become occasions for a prurient speculation which is the opposite of moral imagination. How much did Christ suffer to produce these stains in these unnatural locations? How much did Dax suffer in order to look like this?[5]

The film, at a crucial point in the development of its narrative treatment, whips aside the shroud, so to speak, and shows us Dax before his accident: the whole young man in the various regalias of American male fantasies: the padded figure of the high school football star; the strapped, helmeted figure of the U.S. Air Force pilot; Dax suited, groomed, smiling at his fair prospects. Several of the principals in the film comment on the special tragedy of the accident in that it befell a good-looking young man with an excellent future, as though we need know nothing more about this figure. It is part of the system of conventionalized sentiments that governs such tales that what Dax wants from us—assent to his demand that he should have been allowed to die—cannot be held to have a prehistory.[6] The tone of his demand does not arise out of his character, but out of his accident. Dax's prehistory as Donald Cowart is summed up in images of the typically encumbered American male body.

The male body in America, not least in the small-town, Protestant culture of East Texas where Dax grew up, is not, as is the adolescent female body, a legitimate object of desire. As though to compensate for this repression, however, the flow of attentiveness, of concern, of what an older generation called "spoiling," runs all in one direction between the generations, from parents to children, particularly to sons. It is as though whatever reserves of appetite for life the culture as a whole possesses, its whole tolerance of anarchic animal spirits, of ungoverned will, are projected into the lives of these young men and their typical games. Whether from sublimated desire, or projected rebellion, the culture appears to require the fiction of the giddy desirability of life and of the boundless prospects of the young—in direct denial of the evidence of youthful susceptibility to depression, despair, and nihilism. Can we not imagine that Dax was ever suicidally depressed before his accident? That he was ever petulant about getting his way? That he was ever indulged more than was good for him? We do not know. Would it affect our response to his claim in any case? What does seem clear about the logical structuring of images in the film is that when the massively damaged body, now stark naked, unencumbered with pads and helmets, has allowed us to substitute embarrassed desire with unembarrassed curiosity, we are willing to take the desire to die at face value. We have reached agreement with the young on the question of suicide, but only in the presence of the broken body. There is something about this particular form of suffering, the dashing of these imputed prospects in the young, that permits us to ditch our ordinary social instinct to skepticism. We not only reach agreement with Dax rather too easily; we embrace a dubious notion of consciousness as sincerity and steady purpose, as a way of sealing our agreement with Dax before he eludes us.

V

Leo Braudy's recent book on the history of fame is an account of a central idea in both classical and Christian culture, namely that the self can be fashioned in the light of its need for, and ultimate gratification in, renown.[7] In its long history the idea of fame and the impulse to become famous have taken root in variously defined experiences and opportunities: political and military, civic, literary, spiritual and personal. In our own time, Braudy argues, the idea and the impulse have, as it were, overtaken all possibility of restriction. Fame has become, in Daniel Boorstin's phrase, well-knownness: something sought and achieved for no distinction other than being well known, in itself.[8] Boorstin and Braudy focus on the "marketing" side of fame; theirs is a supply-side reading of renown in which renown is a product of personal experience heightened and amplified first as a feeling of personal distinction and then as a certain kind of cultural product. The perception of personal distinction we may call honor, and the cultural product we may call fame, or renown.

Dax's "case" follows this pattern. His experiences have been interpreted, in the film and in his various retellings, as a conflict of wills over the invasion of his body, of his personal space, of his control over himself, of the rights belonging to his civil personality in a republic. That is, it is a tale of the struggle to retain honor. This struggle is, furthermore, notable; it has brought to the character "Dax" distinction and fame. We have already remarked, at least by implication, how a personal story set out in these terms can only be successfully done so by virtue of cultural conditions over which the "subject" of the story has little or no control: the repression of feeling in the presence of disfigurement; the impoverishment of the public and ritual dimensions of social life; the ideologically motivated fiction of the "accident"; the eagerness to locate the enemy of the moral life in the scientific ethos. Each of these separate issues is telescoped into the presentation of Dax as a man whose experiences, whose honor, whose fame, carry their own authentication. Dax's honor is located strictly within himself and is defined by the story of his struggles.

Consider, however, what happens to this story if we reverse the flow of its central dynamic and take honor and fame to be compensations bestowed by society rather than categories of self-created distinction.

Honor and fame in their classical, predemocratic senses were compensations for the categorical demands of collective codes of behavior. It is worth noting that neither Braudy nor Boorstin in their studies of modern fame notice this possibility. They do not precisely because such a conception of honor is alien to democratic society.

Nevertheless, if we once imaginatively enter into such a possibility it is clear that Dax can receive no honor from the nature of his experiences. In an aristocratic age, these experiences would have placed him in the class of the dishonored—as were the blemished priests at the altars of Jehovah. Honor, in the classical sense, flows not from what arises in personal experience but from the reflexive behavior of an ingrained code exemplified in an individual life. The fame of the person follows from the exemplary character of the life, from the matching of the instance to its model. Dax's story is revealing, therefore, as an instance of a certain kind of pathway to renown that omits the key element of distinction according to the aristocratic principle of honor, namely, a collectively binding principle. The crucial issue here is not the degree of Dax's honesty or courage, or the sincerity of his views, but is the good faith of a society that chooses to attend to Dax by agreeing that he ought to have been allowed to die. Dax's story is properly his own. His fame, however, is a social construction, a conspiracy of agreement, but without a corresponding social bond.

In a democratic society, the mechanisms of compensation cannot have to do with prescribed codes of honor. If they were to apply to Dax at all, in spite of his dishonored condition, we would be saying that under his circumstances, he should have committed suicide. That is, the honorable person would have spared others his apparent dishonor, or, failing that, found a mode of sacrifice that would have lifted his experience into the realm of the mythical. In William Golding's novel *Darkness Visible* the protagonist is a burn victim who lives out his entire life in tragic and eccentric isolation, because of his disfigurement. His life, however, is transfigured in a heroic and sacrificial act of self-immolation. Golding's tale, however, like all his novels, is about natural codes of honor and their consequences for people who uphold them. The elephant man, in Bernard Pomerance's play and in the popular movie, is a man for whom fame had been a degradation; honor was the company of cultivated ladies and gentlemen, whose acceptance of him released in himself a powerful talent for conferring beatitude. Honor had meaning in the context of a Victorian code of class-derived standards of behavior.

These are not the themes of popular American civilization. In America mechanisms of compensation skip honor in these archaic and aristocratic senses altogether. Honor is rather *equivalent* to fame in its contemporary and American sense, as well-knownness. The well-known person is a person compensated for sufferings in a strictly secular sense: He or she enjoys fame while living; it is of no use when dead. Fame/honor is visibly a form of self-aggrandizement, even a form of revenge—as in the film *Prizzi's Honor.* There is a tendency, even in the literature critical of this cultural pattern, to see the personal choices involved as both positive and rational. It is plainly more fun to be famous than not to be famous; the appetite for fame is a natural appetite and need only be balanced by more sober principles of distinction.[9] Dax's case suggests something else, however. Fame as the man-who-should-have-been-allowed-to-die is a throttling compensation—as is perhaps all fame in democratic society, only more so, in that fame outside of the framework of a predetermined code is strictly subject to the dictates of cultural fashion. Fame is the offer we cannot refuse.

There is a theme glanced at in the film, but confined to its weakest possible statement. I mean the theme touched on by Ada Cowart, Dax's mother, when she offered a religious reason for why Dax should not have been allowed to die when his sufferings were greatest. Her reason, that Dax should not have died in his sins, is in fact a very ancient argument of our civilization against suicide or any form of willful death. What should give us pause about Ada Cowart's naive but deeply felt concern is that it represents a powerful cultural agent of comfort and meaning that is out of court for reasons that have nothing to do with Dax's welfare. What if Dax had given his heart to Jesus—as the phrase of old-time religion would have it? Even to ask the question is to peer into that vertiginous American abyss of "choices" that Robert Bellah and his associates turn up again and again in their conversations with thoughtful Americans.[10] All choices seem so terribly arbitrary, so easily translatable into a virtually infinite series of alternatives. What if Dax were a spokesman for a quite different medical/ethical issue than the right to die, say the need for patients to assume their own responsibility for rehabilitation? What if he were a contemplative and a mystic in the fashionable oriental mode? What if he were a country-and-western singer? What if, like the deformed protagonist in Peter Bogdanovich's movie *Mask,* Dax had found community in an outlaw culture, had ridden off with a motorcycle gang? Each of these brings its own constituency, its own rationalizations and rewards, its own degree and context of fame. Our social and civil traditions are silent on what is the good life. They tell us only that we have the right to pursue it.

Most importantly, how do we know what is good for Dax? Can we say merely that he has chosen to see his experiences in the light that he has, and if that is how he wishes to see it we should support him? Yet that is to beg the crucially significant issue of the cultural context in which honor is asserted, choices of identity are confirmed, and fame is sealed. That context is one that trivializes every point of honor, every choice, every ground of fame. To agree with Dax in that context, in whatever measure our agreement colludes with that triviality, is to foreclose on Dax's understanding of his needs, and our understanding of his needs. None of us should wait for a decent society before we can say to a man that we are simply glad he is still with us.

NOTES

1. Michael Ignatieff, *The Needs of Strangers: An Essay on Privacy, Solidarity, and the Politics of Being Human* (London: Chatto & Windus, 1984).

2. Robert J. Lifton, *The Nazi Doctors: Medical Killing and the Psychology of Genocide* (Toronto: Fitzhenry & Whiteside, 1986).

3. An entertaining but rigorous refutation of this tradition is Helen Boss, "A Reappraisal of Marxian Economics: The Productive-Labour Theory of Value and Its Corollaries," *Historical Reflections* 13 (1986): 335ff.

4. The language of costs in relation to human bodies is explored exhaustively and profoundly in Elaine Scarry, *The Body in Pain: The Making and Unmaking of the World* (New York: Oxford University Press, 1985).

5. Georges Didi-Huberman, "The Index of the Absent Wound (Monograph on a Stain)," trans. Thomas Repensek, *October* 29 (Summer 1984): 63–81, is a startling meditation on the Turin shroud. The first subsection of Didi-Huberman's essay is titled "Almost Nothing to See." The system of sentiments invoked by the purely indexical inevitably strip event of its human, storytelling tendency to expansion and elaboration. Among the lunatic efforts at interpreting the shroud that Didi-Huberman records was that of a man who nailed corpses to a cross to see what attitudes produced stains like those on the shroud.

6. A parallel issue is noticed by Michael Howard and Peter Ford, *The True History of the Elephant Man*, rev. ed. (London: Allison and Busby, 1983), 220, in their discussion of previous works on the extraordinary life of Joseph Merrick. Merrick was an extremely disfigured man who had suffered terrible abuse as a circus freak and as a victim of repeated cruelty and betrayal. Ashley Montagu, in *The Elephant Man: A Study in Human Dignity* (London: Allison and Busby, 1972), the book on which Bernard Pomerance's well-known play was based, had noted the problem involved in interpreting the saintly and gentle mature character of Merrick out of a presumption that his previous life was uniformly hellish. Howard and Ford actually uncovered a great deal of information about Merrick's early life, and found that his mature, public self, including his great personal dignity and philosophic and serene temper, in fact had an unsuspected prehistory in a loved and protected early childhood.

7. Leo Braudy, *The Frenzy of Renown: A History of Fame* (New York: Oxford University Press, 1986).

8. Daniel Boorstin, *The Image, Or, What Happened to the American Dream* (New York: Atheneum, 1962).

9. This is the conclusion of Braudy, *Frenzy of Renown*.

10. Robert N. Bellah et al., *Habits of the Heart: Individualism and Commitment in American Life* (Berkeley: University of California Press, 1985).

Dax and Job: The Refusal of Redemptive Suffering

Lonnie D. Kliever

THE RESPONSE OF ORDINARY VIEWERS TO THE film *Dax's Case* is very different from medical and legal professionals, or even from moral and religious philosophers. These technicians and theoreticians of human beatitude are quick to reduce this troubling story about a burn victim's demand to die into a case study in medical ethics or human rights. They press its diverse cast of characters and tragic quest for meaning into neat dichotomies—patient rights vs. medical professionalism, right to die vs. duty to treat, quality of life vs. sanctity of life, autonomous choice vs. paternalistic control. To be sure, these issues are raised in an unforgettable way in this film and they deserve to be debated by all persons who think seriously about problems of informed consent and medical care. But ordinary viewers are beset by very different issues than these "textbook" questions when they ponder *Dax's Case*.

Ordinary people ask questions such as these: "How can anyone understand such absurd accidents? How could anyone endure such senseless suffering? Why must anyone undergo such massive misfortune?" These questions are at once more personal and more universal than the problems raised by the professionals and the philosophers. They go to the very heart of what it means to be a person and to have a world. Indeed, these are the questions that underlie the world's religions. As Clifford Geertz has argued, every religion is an answer to three problems—the problems of intractable bafflement, suffering, and perversity.[1] Human beings and groups cannot long survive in the face of events beyond explanation, of pain beyond relief, of evil beyond repair. The opacity of dumbfounding events, the senselessness of inexorable pain, the enigma of unrequited evil all raise the uncomfortable suspicion that the world, and hence our lives within the world, have no real meaning after all—no dependable regularity, no moral coherence, no transcendent purpose. The religions of humankind respond to these suspicions with pictures of an ordered world and purposeful existence that explain and even celebrate life's ambiguities, inequities, and absurdities.

Seen in this light, the traumatic impact of *Dax's Case* on ordinary people and even trained professionals in their unguarded moments is fully understandable. Dax Cowart's horrifying experience takes us to the very limits of human understanding, endurance, and purpose. The threatening chaos that underlies all of life erupts to the surface in this heartbreaking story of freak accident, disfiguring injury, and menacing despair. *Dax's Case* reminds us that all of the ordinary routines, ordinary capabilities, and ordinary expectations of everyday life can be taken away in one blazing moment of destruction. To be sure, this film confronts us with complicated medical and legal issues, with difficult moral and personal choices. But beneath and beyond these manageable problems lie the *real* questions that beg to be answered—How can we trust a world that can snuff out our lives like a candle? How can we go on living when we wish that we had never been born?

Ultimately, these problems by their very nature do not lend themselves to medical or legal solution. You cannot mend a grieving heart through surgical treatment or create a worthwhile existence by judicial decree. Nor do these problems finally yield to moral or rational analysis. You cannot repair flagrant injustice by moral distinctions or overcome spiritual despair through rational arguments. These technical and theoretical efforts play an important and even indispensable role in human betterment. But there are problems which fall outside their orbits of explanation, amelioration, and transformation. Such problems can only be redressed, if they can be resolved at all, within religion. Religious traditions and systems specialize in those "boundary situations" where persons reach the limits of their analytic capacities, physical endurance, and moral insight. Religions are built to carry the "peak load" of human bafflement, suffering, and perversity.

Thus, the questions that are raised by the film *Dax's Case* are finally and ineluctably religious questions. Indeed, Dax Cowart's experience is a paradigm case of those marginal circumstances which threaten to destroy life's meaning and worth. The burn victim's ordeal of treatment, impairment of function, legacy of disfigurement, limits of rehabilitation, and destruction of relationships are particularly acute expressions of the kinds of trauma that can transform any person's existence into a "living death." Such invasions of chaos into everyday life cannot be repelled or redressed apart from some way of locating the beleaguered individual within a larger universe of meaning and purpose. Religion's role is to secure passage and membership within that "other" world.

I

These deeper religious questions are easily overlooked in *Dax's Case* for at least two reasons. Although the filmmakers were certainly not indifferent to these wider and deeper human issues, they focused their attention on the moral and legal questions arising out of the Cowart story. The primary purpose for this film is educational, and medical, legal, and clerical professionals in training constitute the target audience for this venture. Not surprisingly, the issues raised directly are the moral and legal questions that such professionals will confront in their care of seriously disabled or terminally ill patients.

A second and more important reason why the deeper religious questions may be overlooked lies in the central character of the film. Dax Cowart never addresses his situation, either in prospect or retrospect, from a traditional religious point of view. Cowart appeals to specific legal canons of informed consent, to contemporary social movements for civil rights, and to broad philosophical traditions of personal autonomy in explaining and defending his desires. But he nowhere invokes the Protestant heritage of his culture or the Church of Christ teachings of his childhood to interpret or support his views. Indeed, Cowart's apparent rejection of his own religious heritage goes deeper than either personal modesty about religious commitments or disaffection from religious institutions. Cowart's entire demeanor reflects his own deep alienation from the central symbol and core commitment of the Christian religion. Cowart's approach to his own personal tragedy represents a categorical refusal of *redemptive suffering*.

Every religious tradition—whether ancient or modern, whether Western or Eastern—provides an answer to the enigma of suffering. These religions differ among themselves over whether that answer is an individual or communal undertaking, a human or divine achievement, an earthly or heavenly resolution. Yet every religion offers some way out or some way through the disorder and destruction that seems to haunt all of human life. Every religion offers a way to relieve suffering, including the suffering of death, from sheer randomness and senselessness. Moreover, all the so-called "world" or "higher" religions endorse some version of the way of *redemptive* suffering—of suffering for the sake of some larger social or some higher spiritual good. For example, the Christian tradition carries the principle of redemptive suffering into the very heart of its understanding of divine as well as human life. The symbol of the crucified and resurrected Christ—at once both fully human and fully divine—points to suffering's deepest mystery and ultimate resolution. God and humankind undergo suffering together in order to break the grip of evil and to deprive the grave of victory over this world. Or again, the Hindu tradition swallows up all of the perceived dualities of spirit and matter, creation and destruction, pleasure and pain in one great Everlasting Unity. Whether through the yogic way of knowledge, work, devotion, or meditation, the promise and goal of the Hindu path to redemption is total immersion in this great Cosmic Dance of Life and Death.

We search in vain for any echo of such redemptive suffering in Dax Cowart's approach to his own pain and death. He nowhere sees his accident as an occasion for deepening his spiritual relationship to God. He nowhere confronts his pain as the supreme test of his faith in the face of adversity. He nowhere resolves to conquer his handicaps to help others facing similar circumstances. He nowhere defends his attempted suicides as an effort to relieve others of the burden of his care. Others in the film voice these possibilities for him. Cowart's mother, Ada, prays that he will live long enough to come back to God. His physician, Duane Larson, dares Cowart to be man enough to accept the challenge of living with pain. Cowart's lawyer, Rex Houston, encourages him to use the money he has to make something of his life. His friend, Art Rousseau, observes that Cowart has good reasons for wanting to end his life. But Dax reaches out for none of these traditional ways of redeeming his own suffering from utter waste and despair.

II

In and of itself, Dax's refusal of redemptive suffering may not signal a categorical rejection of *religious* commitments and consolations. There are, after all, older archaic and aristocratic religious traditions which offered no promises and made no demands of *redemptive* suffering. In archaic religions, as exemplified in the Gilgamesh Epic of ancient Babylon, pain and death are brute facts of human existence which resist all efforts at penultimate relief or ultimate resolution. Gilgamesh's frantic search for an answer to the problem of suffering is disappointed at every turn. Siduri's efforts to dissuade him from his fruitless quest finally proved wise and true:

> Gilgamesh, where are you running?
> You will not find the immortal life you seek.
> When the gods created man

191

They ordained death for man
And kept immortality for themselves.
Make merry day and night.
Make every day a day of joy.
Dance, play, day and night.
Wear dazzling clothes,
Bathe your head. Refresh yourself with water.
Cherish the child who grasps your hand.
Let your wife rejoice in your bosom.
For this is the fate of man.[2]

The only "answer" to pain and death is to live life fully while you have the health and the wealth to enjoy it.

By contrast, certain aristocratic religious traditions, such as the Samurai Code of the premodern Japanese ruling class, regarded pain and death as "lighter than a feather."[3] The legendary suicidal courage and martial skill of these warriors who dominated Japanese society for seven hundred years were most often brought into play in wars of defense and conquest. But beyond and beneath their willingness to suffer and die for the sake of their masters and their tribes, the samurai lived by a code of personal honor more important than mere loyalty or even life itself. *Bushido,* the chivalric way of the warrior, embraced extreme suffering as the ultimate badge of such personal integrity. Not surprisingly, *bushido's* ultimate expression was *seppuku,* the formal name for the rite of *hara-kiri* meaning "cutting of the belly." This excruciatingly painful form of suicide was the prerogative of the samurai class alone. Only the elite warrior class were required to display their unique personal courage and determination by undergoing this agonizing ordeal. As such, for the samurai, ultimately pain and death served no larger or higher good beyond the demonstration of one's own inner sincerity and integrity.

But there are religious resources closer at hand than these archaic or aristocratic traditions for those like Dax Cowart who cannot and will not embrace the principle of redemptive suffering. In fact, there are within the canonical texts of Judaism and Christianity subversive alternatives to the very idea that suffering serves some larger social or higher spiritual good. These alternatives are clearly in evidence in the Bible's so-called "Wisdom Literature." Certain of the Psalms and Proverbs, but especially the books of Ecclesiastes and Job contain echoes of an archaic evasion or an aristocratic embrace of unrequited suffering which are completely at odds with the Bible's prevailing view of suffering. Indeed, the stories of Job and Dax contain narrative elements that are hauntingly similar. Both suffer calamities that strip them of everything but life itself. Both beg eloquently for death's deliverance to no avail. Both contend with "comforters" who seek to explain away their plight. Both resume life again beyond their terrible pain and loss. But the similarities between Job's "lament" and Dax's "case" go deeper than mere structural affinities. There are thematic similarities at the very heart of their stories. Rightly understood, Job's story no less than Dax's represents a categorical refusal of redemptive suffering.

III

To be sure, the Book of Job in its canonical version seems to offer a ringing confirmation of the principle of redemptive suffering. This ancient prince was showered with heavenly favor and earthly success. Job had a beautiful wife and family, thousands of sheep and camels, hundreds of oxen and asses. Job enjoyed the devotion of his many servants and the admiration of his many subjects. Best of all, Job basked in the attentive love and care of his God. But one day that divine love and care was called into question for both God and Job. God had been boasting to his celestial court about Job:

> Have you considered my servant Job, that there is none like him on the earth, a blameless and upright man, who fears God and turns away from evil? (1 : 8)[4]

Then Satan, God's ancient Adversary, called the Lord's hand:

> Does Job fear God for nought? Hast thou not put a hedge about him and his house and all that he has, on

193

every side? Thou hast blessed the work of his hands, and his possessions have increased in the land. But put forth thy hand now, and touch all that he has, and he will curse thee to thy face. (1:9–11)

So the lines were drawn between God and Satan, between good and evil, with Job as the centerpiece in this cosmic struggle.

In rapid and bewildering succession, Job suffered every grief and loss known to humankind. Enemy forces wiped out his servants and livestock. Natural disasters destroyed his home and children. Yet Job did not renounce his faith:

> Naked I came from my mother's womb, and naked
> I shall return; the Lord gave, and the Lord has taken
> away; blessed be the name of the Lord. (1:21)

Then new woes came striking Job's flesh and breaking his heart. Job was afflicted with loathsome sores from head to toe that filled him with misery and revolted others with disgust. After a time, even his wife could no longer stand the sight and sense of his suffering. She walked out on him, advising Job to give up on his faith in God and let go of his hold on life. Even his friends who came to comfort him spent their time trying to convince Job that he was somehow to blame for the terrible disasters that had befallen him. Still Job did not compromise his integrity:

> As God lives, who has taken away my right,
>   and the Almighty, who has made my soul bitter;
> as long as my breath is in me,
>   and the spirit of God is in my nostrils;
> my lips will not speak falsehood,
>   and my tongue will not utter deceit. (27:1–4)

Job remained faithful to God in the face of the loss of everything— houses and lands, family and friends, health and happiness, meaning and purpose.

Having thus been vindicated against the slurs of Satan, God

was free to return Job to earthly prosperity and heavenly favor. Since Job had shown that his devotion to God was not "bought" by God's benevolence, he could be trusted with all of the riches of health and happiness that once were his. In fact, the Lord gave Job twice as much as he had before. Job's kinsmen and subjects returned to his house bearing gifts and showing sympathy. He recultivated his lands and rebuilt his herds. He reestablished his family and was given seven strong sons and three beautiful daughters. Best of all, he lived long enough to see four generations of his descendants. Finally Job died peacefully and naturally, "an old man, and full of days."

Though good triumphs over evil in the end in this ancient tale, many contemporary readers are troubled by the way this monumental struggle is portrayed. There is a certain theological crudity and credulity about the whole affair, particularly the brief prose prologue and conclusion which frames the poetic body of the story which details Job's conversations with God and his friends. God appears to be anything but a heavenly *Father!* For the sake of winning a wager over a cynic in the heavenly council, the Deity allows his favorite servant to be tortured by excruciating pain and loss. Surely Job's suffering—to say nothing of the death of his innocent children and his hapless servants—was an intolerable exercise of the divine prerogative and power. And what about Job's surprising failure of nerve at the end of the story? For all of his protested innocence against his three "comforters" and for all of his bitter demands that God explain his terrible afflictions, in the end Job grovels before the unfathomable mystery of the Universe.

Little wonder that Robert Frost, in *A Masque of Reason*, pokes fun at God for his heavenly duplicity and at Job for his earthly complicity:

> GOD I'm going to tell Job why I tortured him
> And I trust it won't be adding to the torture.
> I was just showing off to the Devil, Job,
> As is set forth in chapters One and Two.

(Job takes a few steps pacing.) Do you mind?
(God eyes him anxiously.)

JOB   No. No, I mustn't.
'Twas human of You. I expected more
Than I could understand and what I get
Is almost less than I can understand.
But I don't mind. Let's leave it as it stood.
The point was it was none of my concern.
I stick to that.[5]

On the face of things, Job's God seems too capricious and God's Job too compliant for our modern tastes in either divinity or humanity. We are no happier with a man who offers self-immolation as the pledge of his faith than with a God who demands self-abasement as the price of his love.

But these latter-day objections are the product of an overly *literal* reading of the canonical story of Job. Taking the story as a whole, the book of Job totally rejects all theories of suffering as divine punishment for human sin. To be sure, punitive theories of suffering are ancient and enduring because they have a certain plausibility and undeniable power. Empirically, a great deal of pain and sorrow can be laid at the door of willful ignorance and human perversity. We do bring much suffering on ourselves and on others by acts of wanton carelessness and selfishness. Existentially, the idea that suffering is a punishment for sin at least frees evil from sheer caprice and absurdity. We can at least find some meaning in our afflictions if they are sent by God to chastise the wicked and to confirm the virtuous. But, for all of that according to the Book of Job, punitive theories of suffering simply do not plumb the heights of divine mystery or the depths of human misery.

What more dramatic way of undercutting theories of punitive suffering than through a case study of suffering wholly undeserved? Job's complete innocence is the essential precondition of the dramatic action of the Joban story and each narrative element of the story serves that end. God's gratuitous wager with Satan confirms that Job suffered through no personal or collective fault. Neither Job, nor kinsman nor countrymen brought these baleful disasters upon his head. Job's well-meaning friends serve as the dramatic foil against which both Job and God contend. Eliphaz, Bildad, and Zophar argue every side of the punitive approach to human misery. Eliphaz insists that human standards of justice cannot be applied to the divine purpose. Bildad insists that God's justice forecloses all debate about whether human beings suffer necessarily for cause. Zophar drives the argument home by insisting that human wickedness deserves even worse punishments than God allows to befall the sinner. But Job will not be browbeaten by his three "comforters" and stoutly maintains his integrity against their charges. He even carries his case to God himself, bitterly protesting his undeserved agony and demanding that God show him his iniquities and transgressions. But God never replies to the demand that he show cause for Job's suffering, since there were no justifiable reasons for his afflictions in the first place. Indeed, God showers his blessings upon Job only when Job stops asking for a justification of his suffering and simply accepts God's power over everything that exists and everything that happens in the universe.

In other words, the canonical Book of Job is not a story about how to *explain* suffering but about how to *redeem* suffering. Whatever its origins and deserts, suffering can only be overcome by trusting in God to bring some good purpose and final ending to suffering. That trust is what brought forth the outpouring of blessings upon Job once he has proven God right against the sneers and dares of Satan! Job is not rewarded for his *suffering,* as if somehow suffering restored the moral balance of the universe or satisfied the wrath of an angry God. Job is rewarded for his *faithfulness,* by his willingness to trust in God even at the cost of horrendous suffering by himself and those he loved. Thus, for all of the theological and moral naivete of its plot, the story of Job presents a sublime view of redemptive suffering. Not only does the story of Job proclaim that all suffering can finally be redeemed from absurdity, but it also leaves room for the possibility that both God and Humankind are involved in that ultimate transformation—a possibility eventually made explicit in the Christian tradition's symbol of the Cross of Christ.

IV

Having said all that, there is an alternative reading of the story of Job that presents a complete break with the principle of *redemptive* suffering. Literary analysis of the Book of Job in its present canonical form shows that it is not the work of a single author. Rather, it comes from a school of ancient storytellers, poets, sages, and scribes who worked over materials stretching back half a millenium or more. Such "sociological authorship" was the rule rather than the exception in ancient Semitic cultures. Even today among Bedouin nomads, tribal storytellers draw on a repertoire of ancient songs and proverbs, myths and poems in spinning stories of inspiration and instruction for their tribal group. Thus, the Book of Job as we have it in the Jewish and Christian canons of Holy Scripture is a product of diverse oral and literary traditions that passed through many recensions in reaching its final form.

Any detailed reconstruction of the growth of the story of Job is a matter of some conjecture.[6] But most contemporary biblical scholars agree that the Book of Job is not *a* book but *two* books, or rather a magnificent poem encased by an artless prose introduction and conclusion. Moreover, the shorter prose narrative obviously comes from a very different period and presents a very different theology than the much longer poetic dialogues which constitute the body of the Joban epic. Biblical scholars disagree among themselves over whether the story or the poem came first. Some say the story was an ancient folktale of heroic faith that served as the literary inspiration for a later philosophical reflection on human misery, written in the form of poetic dialogues. Other scholars see the poem as an early gnomic meditation on human suffering which was later placed in the more "orthodox" mythological framework of a contest between God and Satan. On either reconstruction, the notion of *redemptive*

suffering belongs to the prose narrative rather than to the poetic dialogues of Job.

Stripped of its mythological beginning and ending, the poetic
dialogues of Job proffer no final resolution to suffering whether in
this life or in some life to come. Indeed, this austere poetic vision of
human misery is advocated in the teeth of the traditional view of
divine retribution and rewards. Job's colloquy with his three "comforters" is a brilliant deconstruction of any and all notions that God
sends suffering either for human punishment or for human betterment. Eliphaz, Bildad, and Zophar did their best to convince Job
that his suffering must be deserved since the world is governed by a
divine law that always rewards the good and punishes the wicked.
They piled up reason upon reason drawn from observed experience,
ancient tradition, and esoteric wisdom, but Job countered their insistent claims at every turn. Of course, Job had greater tact than to
attack their fundamental presuppositions directly, but he subtly un-
dermined the traditional notion of divine law by insisting on his
own innocence. What he knew of his own sufferings and what he
could see of the world's sufferings bore no direct relation to individual or collective guilt.

Therein lay Job's greatest agony. His cry for death was not a
plea for release from a life of physical misery so much as a protest of
despair against a life devoid of spiritual meaning. Little wonder that
he turned from the debate with his friends to the debate with God.
He finally carried his misgivings about cosmic justice before the
heavenly tribunal where he stoutly defended his innocence and de-
fiantly called God to account:

> Oh, that I had one to hear me!
> (Here is my signature! let the Almighty answer
> me!)
> Oh, that I had the indictment written by my
> adversary!
> Surely I would carry it on my shoulder;

I would bind it on me as a crown;
I would give him an account of all my steps;
    like a prince I would approach him.
"If my land has cried out against me,
    and its furrows have wept together;
if I have eaten its yield without payment,
    and caused the death of its owners;
let thorns grow instead of wheat, and foul weeds instead
    of barley." (31:35–40)

Line upon line, strophe upon strophe, Job demanded justice from God but God remained silent—neither convincing him of his sin nor delivering him from his suffering.

At last God answered Job out of the whirlwind, but still there were no explanations or resolutions of his suffering. Instead, God confronted Job with a universe beyond his comprehension and control. Has Job "entered into the springs of the sea" or "cleft a channel for the torrents of rain?" Can Job "bind the chains of the Pleiades" or "draw out Leviathan with a fishhook?" Did Job "give the horse his might" or "make the ground to put forth grass?" Power upon power, glory upon glory, God piles up the sheer majesty and magnitude of life, culminating in that terrible challenge for Job to "gird up your loins *like a man*":

Deck yourself with majesty and dignity;
    clothe yourself with glory and splendor.
Pour forth the overflowings of your anger,
    and look on every one that is proud, and abase
    him.
Look on everyone that is proud, and bring him low;
    and tread down the wicked where they stand.
Hide them all in the dust together;
    bind their faces to the world below.
Then will I also acknowledge to you,
    that your own right hand can give you victory.
    (40:10–14)

Whereupon Job repented of his rage against life's inequity and God's indifference. End of poem—no miraculous recoveries of health and wealth, no miraculous returns of family and friends! Only the challenge to go on living a just and decent life in spite of everything.

The poem could have no other ending. To the old poet or poets who wrote this drama thousands of years ago, the injustice of the universe was self-evident. Job's sufferings—and they were meant to be the most dreadful sufferings imaginable—were never justified. In the final analysis, Job's sufferings were not attributable to human sin or amenable to divine grace. Yet, though Job's bitter protest against the injustice of his sufferings explained nothing, his agonizing inquiry into the meaning of his life changed everything! The irony is that Job had no reason to live until he gave up on his demands for cosmic justice. Job knew that, if a person gets what he deserves in life, he was being cheated—cheated so badly that he had no other recourse but to curse God and choose death! But, once Job saw through the "mangy miracle" of life, he was able to go on with his own life in spite of his pain and loss.

What Job learned out of his encounter with the terrifying and creative energy of the universe is that human beings are one another's only hope. Job lost everything that human beings cherish— wealth and health, family and friends, dignity and purpose. As each layer of life's meaning was peeled away, Job had less and less reason for going on with his life. But, when he reached the bottom of his fortunes, he made the great human discovery. He discovered that, whatever else he was, he was a human being. He could still ask questions of the universe. He could still demand answers of the universe. What more exquisite image of the fundamental irony of the human situation can be imagined? Job sitting alone on the dung heap, in his rags, covered with boils, receiving life's answer to his bitter questions and belligerent demands: "Deck *yourself* with majesty and dignity! Your *own* right hand can give you victory!" The only answer to life's problems is found in the human capacity to live life over and over again, whatever the pain and whenever the peril.

V

This humanistic "reading" of Job's story has been given powerful contemporary expression in Archibald MacLeish's verse drama, entitled *J. B.*[7] Curiously enough, MacLeish makes use of the whole canonical story of Job in spelling out his own humanistic vision of human suffering. MacLeish's play within a play takes place under a circus tent. Two broken-down actors named Zuss and Nickles, reduced to selling popcorn and balloons at the circus, don the masks of God and Satan left behind and stage their version of a drama that is played out at each performance under the big top. J. B. is a wealthy and successful banker enjoying the blessings of heaven and earth. Suddenly all these blessings are taken away from him in a shattering succession of Joban catastrophes—his soldier son slain after an armistice had been declared, his teenage son and daughter mangled in an automobile crash, his youngest child raped and murdered by a psychopath, his surviving daughter and accumulated wealth destroyed in a bombing that leveled the entire town, his body reduced to suppurating sores, his wife driven away by despair and disgust. With Zuss pontificating and Nickles kibitzing, J. B. plays out the drama of his desperate struggle to find the meaning of these unexpurgated horrors.

Foreshadowing his humanistic sensibilities, MacLeish reverses all the plot lines in the Joban story. In a brilliant twist, J. B. protests his guilt rather than his innocence against his three "comforters," who are portrayed as spokesmen for the three major deterministic ideologies in our culture. Bildad, a Marxist historian, argues that suffering is a by-product of class conflict and guilt is a "sociological accident." Eliphaz, a Freudian psychoanalyst, counsels that suffering is a consequence of neurotic repression and guilt is a "psychophenomenal situation." Zophar, a Calvinistic theologian, proclaims that suffering is a result of original sin and guilt is a "deceptive secret." But J. B. refuses these blandishments of individual impotence, even while insisting that his own crimes deserve nothing like the sufferings inflicted on him:

> I'd rather suffer
> Every unspeakable suffering God sends,
> Knowing that it was I that suffered,
> I that had earned the need to suffer,
> I that acted, I that chose,
> Than wash my hands with yours in that
> Defiling innocence. Can we be men
> And make an irresponsible ignorance
> Responsible for everything? I will not
> Listen to you![8]

For J. B., the elimination of individual guilt would make the whole world meaningless, since it would destroy all possibility of individual freedom and moral responsibility.

MacLeish gives an even more startling reversal to the end of J. B.'s struggle to find the meaning of his suffering. As in the canonical story, J. B. gets back twice over everything he has lost at the end of the play. Yet, for MacLeish, the wonder of that ending is not that God *gives* everything back but that Job *takes* everything back! After J. B. is finally reduced to abnegation and repentance by the silence of the universe, Nickles sneers that human beings always end up broken in body and spirit—"Pious, contemptible, goddam sheep/Without the spunk to spit on Christmas!" Quickly, Zuss reminds Nickles that there is always one more scene. No matter who plays "Job" or how he plays it, he "gets all he ever had and more—much more." But Nickles snorts at the very thought:

> Live his life again?—
> Not even the most ignorant, obstinate,
> Stupid or degraded man
> This filthy planet ever farrowed,
> Offered the opportunity to live
> His bodily life twice over, would accept it—
> Least of all Job, poor, trampled bastard![9]

Any man "screwed as Job was" would rather "reject the whole creation with a stale pink pill" than live his life again. To Nickles's astonishment, however, J. B. takes up his life again. The man once highest and happiest who had suffered every anguish and loss—whose property had been swept away by disaster, whose children had been killed by chance, whose body had become a running sore, whose wife had deserted him in disgust, whose pleas for death went unheeded, whose demands for justice were ignored—that man *accepts* his life again! J. B. starts life over again—falls in love again, goes to work again—facing the same risks of pain and loss all over again!

J. B.'s decision to take up his life again has nothing to do with God. All the traditional comforts and consolations of his religion were called into question by the holocaust of pain and loss that he had undergone. Indeed, J. B.'s agonizing struggle with the massive injustice and indifference of the universe had shattered his faith in God as a miraculous problem solver and benevolent need fulfiller. J. B.'s story ends on a dark and bare stage. Zuss and Nickles are seen and heard no more. J. B. is utterly alone amid the rubble of his home and his world. Suddenly his wife Sarah appears out of the darkness, a sprig of forsythia in her hand. They talk about what had pulled them apart—J. B.'s futile longing for justification and Sarah's futile looking for escape. Neither way of dealing with their tragedy had worked, leaving them nothing but one another in the face of utter despair. They embrace warmly and then begin straightening up the tumbled furniture remaining in the room. At last, reminiscent of Nietzsche's vision of a world without God, Sarah voices the truth born out of their terrible pain and loss:

> Blow on the coal of the heart.
> The candles in churches are out.
> The lights have gone out in the sky.
> Blow on the coal of the heart
> And we'll see by and by . . .[10]

Finally, there are no answers to human suffering other than the answers found in human work and human love.

VI

Whether couched in ancient verse or staged in modern drama, Job's story is relevant to every age since, in MacLeish's words, "there's always someone playing Job." Nickles puts it bitterly but accurately:

> Job is everywhere we go,
> His children dead, his work for nothing,
> Counting his losses, scraping his boils,
> Discussing himself with his friends and physicians,
> Questioning everything—the times, the stars,
> His own soul, God's providence.[11]

Millions and billions since time began have found themselves in Job's shoes. But no one in our time has "played Job" more powerfully and hauntingly than Dax Cowart!

As noted above, the narrative parallels between Job's and Dax's stories are obvious upon a moment's reflection. Both are fairhaired boys with brilliant futures—Job with his riches and his fame, Dax with his good looks and his abilities. Both are innocent victims of unspeakable calamities—Job with his plundered realm and pustulant body, Dax with his sightless world and scarred flesh. Both are eloquent protesters against life's injustice—Job with his demand that God show him his iniquity, Dax with his plea that he be allowed to die. Both are hapless recipients of well-meaning "comforters"—Job with his counselors who urged him to shoulder the blame for his plight, Dax with his caretakers who compelled him to carry the burden of his life. Both are prosperous survivors of harrowing ordeals—Job with his redoubled riches and rebuilt family, Dax with his litigated wealth and solicitous helpers. The plot lines of Dax's story seem almost borrowed from those of Job's, as if all stories of human suffering are but versions of a single archetype.

Moreover, as suggested earlier, the structural symmetries between Dax's and Job's stories go much deeper than narrative detail, particularly if we separate Job's story from its "orthodox" theological framework. Dax is no more willing than Job, or his modern counterpart J. B., to settle for a *redemptive* explanation of his sufferings. Against his caretakers during those long months of hospital treatment, Dax resisted all entreaties from physicians and advisors, all efforts by family and friends to turn his sufferings into some larger good. We listen in vain to the recounting of that time in his life by Dax and others for some telltale evidence that Dax finally embraced his sufferings as an occasion for spiritual growth, heroic courage, exemplary achievement, or even stoic endurance. Nor is Dax any more disposed today to accept the idea that his sufferings have been thus redeemed by subsequent developments in his life. His mother points to Dax's business and marriage as justification for the continuation of her son's treatment. His physicians, Charles Baxter, Robert Meier, Duane Larson, and Robert White, point out how much they have learned from Dax about caring for the disabled and the dying. His lawyer and friend, Rex Houston, expresses pride in Dax's efforts to gain a law degree and to become a businessman. These later developments have more than justified Dax's sufferings in the eyes of those who ignored his pleas to die and gave him the chance to live. But, if we take Dax at his word, none of these developments has redeemed his sufferings in his *own* eyes! Dax still maintains his protest against his sufferings and those who allowed those sufferings to continue: "If the same thing were to occur tomorrow and, knowing that I could reach this point, I would still not want to be forced to undergo the pain and agony that I had to undergo to be alive now." [12]

VII

Herein lies the pathos of Dax's story when compared to Job's. Unlike ancient Job, or his modern counterpart J. B., Dax has not reached a clearly positive alternative to the scheme of redemptive suffering he rejects. He seems to define his existence more by negation than by affirmation, more by death than by life. Looking back on his months of treatment, Dax remains embittered against his family and physicians for their refusals to let him die. His recollections of those terrible months in the hospital still sound like the words of those who have suffered unspeakable agonies at the hands of uncaring tormentors. His treatment was "as painful as being boiled in hot oil." All he could do was "scream at the top of my lungs until I passed out from exhaustion." In the final analysis, "I was nothing more than a hostage to the current state of medical technology. If the explosion had occurred only two or three years earlier, I would have died. But, simply because the state of the art had changed, I did not die and I was forced to receive treatment." Looking forward to his years of survival, Dax remains tentative about his commitment to life. He grudgingly admits that he "enjoys life now" and that "it feels good to be alive." But he worries about the possibility that the "quality of his life" might once again become intolerable: "For instance, in my case, if I were to lose my hearing—I could not listen to music, read books, talk with people, any number of things I enjoy now—I feel that I would have an unacceptable quality of life at that point." Caught between bemoaning his survival and begrudging his existence, Dax remains torn between life and death.

Of course, Dax had and has every reason to prefer death over life. Beyond the temporary pain of his treatments was the permanent pain of his impairments. Radically disfigured and severely maimed, Dax was permanently robbed of abilities and sensibilities that are simply taken for granted by able-bodied and competent adults. He lived for years with the humiliation of others feeding and toileting him like an overgrown infant. He struggled with the aversion of others pitying and avoiding him like a sideshow freak. To be sure, Dax in recent years has achieved a remarkable level of personal independence and social adjustment. He has created a private and public life for himself that has brought him personal satisfaction and social recognition. But even these remarkable achievements have brought no "happy ending" to his story. Both the business he established and the marriage he entered during the film-ing of *Dax's Case* have subsequently failed. He still confronts daily the elemental fears that have haunted him from his earliest days in the hospital—that he could never do anything but "sell pencils on the street corner" and that he would never "establish a relationship with a member of the opposite sex." Little wonder that Dax might greet each new day asking whether the game is worth the candle after all. Where is the meaning of any human life deprived of pro-ductive work and responsive love?

But Dax's fixation on the dark side of his life is maintained by deeper reserves than his massive physical handicaps and chronic psychological apprehensions. Dax is locked into an essentially nega-tive outlook on life by two powerful mythologies which, like all "story-shaped" systems of reality formation and personality defini-tion, have deeply conditioned his sense of the world and his place in the world. On the one hand, Dax is heir to a *public mythology* that celebrates the good life which now eludes him. What Erich Fromm has called the "marketing orientation" dominates the modern under-standing of human nature and human relationships.[13] Human life is a competitive market where success is more the result of looks and personality than of skill and character. This principal of evaluation applies the same to both human relationships and human activities. Love and work alike are commodities whose worth depends upon their exchange value. In a world defined by this marketing orien-tation, Dax is "damaged goods" in the most literal sense of the word—a fact that the film *Dax's Case* brings home with brutal can-dor in its segued images of horrific treatment scenes and family al-bum flashbacks. Dax's exchange value will never count for much on the commodity markets of either modern work or modern love.

On the other hand, Dax is heir to a *private mythology* that com-memorates the "good death" that was denied him. No one can be surprised that Dax's story of his plea to die plays a pivotal role in his life. Life-threatening events are often life-changing events, doubly so when those past experiences permanently mark a person the way Dax's accident and treatment did. Under normal circumstances, people who have undergone some harrowing experience are able to "rework" their stories as they gain distance and perspective on the meaning of that experience. But Dax's "editing" abilities are limited by the fact that he told his story of pain in an unforgettable way in the videotape *Please Let me Die* during his treatment in 1974 at Galveston's John Sealy Hospital. That videotape made Dax a legendary figure in medical and legal circles concerned with issues of death and dying. He became "The Man Who Was Sentenced to Life." [14] That legendary status has grown even larger with the film *Dax's Case* and through the public appearances and media attention which it has generated. Dax has become "The Man Who Lives to Defend the Right to Die." [15] Little wonder that Dax is deeply invested in maintaining this image of himself, since it finally brought him the sense of personal worth and public recognition he so desperately needed. But, maintaining that image has cost him the freedom to embrace his life now, lest he thereby "prove" that his family and physicians were right after all in refusing to let him die.

Torn between a life he cannot achieve and a death he was denied, Dax seems fully committed to neither living nor dying. There are alternatives to the public and private mythologies which leave Dax pulled between life and death. The most obvious alternatives are those offered by the traditional religions, with their promise of divine deliverance from sufferings borne for the sins of the world or for the glory of God. But, for reasons which are evident though not explained, Dax will have none of these. Dax apparently has little interest in blaming or blessing God for the horrors he has endured. Still there are other nontraditional religious alternatives available, none more appropriate to Dax's past experiences and present needs than the ancient wisdom of Job. The "absurd heroism" of Job offers Dax a mythic pattern for affirming his life without trivializing its tragedy. Job's story undercuts optimistic and cynical worldviews alike. Job holds out no promises for ultimate success and happiness and hands down no counsels of utter failure and despair. Rather, Job reveals that human sufferings and human satisfactions are as inseparable as they are inexhaustible. Holding those twin fates in balance without concealing life's absurdity or relinquishing life's heroism is the fundamental task facing every human being who has ever lived.

As things stand, Dax has not yet learned the whole of Job's truth. He surely has tasted of the world—"licked the stick that beat his brains out." He has seen human life through to the very bottom. He remains convinced that nothing on earth can ever *redeem* the human condition. But Dax has not yet forgiven the world—"taken the seed up of the sad creation, planting the hopeful world again." He has not affirmed human life out to the very end. He remains dubious that nothing on earth can ever *exhaust* the human prospect. But Dax's own inherent honesty and courage may yet bring him to Job's final verdict on this hideous and heartless world:

> Blow on the coal of the heart.
> The candles in churches are out.
> The lights have gone out in the sky.
> Blow on the coal of the heart
> And we'll see by and by . . .

Should he attain that ancient wisdom, Dax would become the complete hero for all those who sooner or later must "play Job." He would thereby confer and confirm on all the suffering sons and daughters of earth the will to live as well as the right to die!

NOTES

1. Clifford Geertz, *The Interpretations of Cultures* (New York: Basic Books, 1973), 101–8.

2. Gilgamesh Epic cited in Gerald A. Larue, *Ancient Myth and Modern Life* (Long Beach: Center Line Press, 1988), 88–89.

3. Richard Storry and Werner Forman, *The Way of the Samurai* (London: Orbis Publishing, 1978), 29–33.

4. All citations from the Book of Job are from the *Revised Standard Version of the Bible* (New York: National Council of Churches, 1952).

5. Robert Frost, *A Masque of Reason* (New York: Henry Holt and Company, 1945), 16–17.

6. For a summary of the many hypotheses of the composition of the Book of Job, see Samuel Terrien, "Introduction and Exegesis of the Book of Job," *The Interpreter's Bible*, III (New York and Nashville: Abingdon Press, 1954), 877ff.

7. Archibald MacLeish, *J. B.: A Play in Verse* (Boston: Houghton Mifflin Company, 1958).

8. Ibid., 123.

9. Ibid., 143–44.

10. Ibid., 153.

11. Ibid., 13.

12. All citations from the film, *Dax's Case*, Concern for Dying, Inc., New York, 1985.

13. Erich Fromm, *Man for Himself* (New York: Rinehart and Company, Inc., 1947), 67–82.

14. Ken Lanterman, "The Life Sentence of Dax Cowart," *Houston Post*, February 8, 1987, 1G, 6G.

15. Toni Giovanetti, "The Trials of Dax," *Dallas Times Herald*, April 10, 1986, 1D, 4–5D.

Dax's Case is available for rental or purchase in 16 mm film and 1/2" or 3/4" videocassette from

Filmakers Library
124 East 40th Street
New York, New York 10016
(212) 355-6545

or

Concern for Dying
250 West 57th Street
New York, New York 10107
(800) 248-2122
(212) 246-6962

Notes on Contributors

Keith Burton is the vice president of Hill and Knowlton, Inc., a public relations firm in Dallas, Texas.

Courtney C. Campbell, Ph.D., is associate editor of the *Hastings Center Report* and resides in Carmel, New York.

James F. Childress, Ph.D., is Kyle Professor of Religious Studies and professor of medical education at the University of Virginia in Charlottesville, Virginia.

H. Tristram Engelhardt, Jr., Ph.D., M.D., is professor in the Departments of Medicine and Community Medicine and in the Center for Ethics, Medicine, and Public Issues at Baylor College of Medicine in Houston, Texas.

Sally Gadow, Ph.D., is associate professor in the Institute for the Medical Humanities of the University of Texas Medical Branch in Galveston, Texas.

Stanley Johannesen, Ph.D., is associate professor of history at the University of Waterloo in Ontario, Canada.

Patricia A. King, J.D., is associate professor of law at Georgetown University Law Center in Washington, D.C.

Lonnie D. Kliever, Ph.D., is professor of religious studies at Southern Methodist University in Dallas, Texas.

Joanne Lynn, M.D., is associate director of ICU Research at the George Washington University Medical Center in Washington, D.C.

William F. May, Ph.D., is Cary M. Maguire University Professor of Ethics at Southern Methodist University in Dallas, Texas.

William J. Winslade, Ph.D., J. D., is professor of medical jurisprudence and psychiatry at the Institute for the Medical Humanities of the University of Texas Medical Branch in Galveston, Texas.

Robert B. White, M.D., is Marie B. Gale Professor of Psychiatry at the University of Texas Medical Branch in Galveston, Texas.

Richard M. Zaner, Ph.D., is Ann Geddes Stahlman Professor of Medical Ethics at the Vanderbilt University School of Medicine in Nashville, Tennessee.

Index